Mental Health and Mental Illness

Mental Health and Mental Illness

A Workbook for General Nurse Students

Wendy Nganasurian RMN SRN RNT

Tutor, RMN Postregistration Course
West Essex School of Nursing
St Margaret's Hospital
Epping, Essex

An H M + M Nursing publication
JOHN WILEY & SONS
Chichester · New York · Brisbane · Toronto · Singapore

H M + M Publishers is an imprint of John Wiley & Sons Ltd

Library of Congress Cataloging-in-Publication Data:

Nganasurian, Wendy.
    Mental health and mental illness: a workbook for general
nurse students/Wendy Nganasurian.
       p. cm—(Nursing modules series) (An H M + M nursing
publication)
    Includes bibliographies and index.
    ISBN 0 471 91972 1
    1. Psychiatric nursing. 2. Mental illness. 3. Mental health.
I. Title. II. Series: H M + M nursing modules series.
III. Series: An H M + M nursing publication.
    [DNLM: 1. Mental Health—nurses' instruction.
2. Psychiatric Nursing. WY 160 N576m]
RC440.N43 1988
610.73'68—dc19
DNLM/DLC
for Library of Congress

British Library Cataloguing in Publication Data

Nganasurian, Wendy
  Mental health and mental illness.
  1. Man. Mental disorders—For nursing
  I. Title   II. Series
  616.89'0024613

  ISBN 0 471 91972 1

Phototypeset by Dobbie Typesetting Service, Plymouth, Devon
Printed by Anchor Brendon Ltd., Tiptree, Colchester.

Contents

Preface

This workbook has been written specifically to provide general nursing students with a clear and concise introduction to the care of patients experiencing mental health problems, whether in the general ward setting or during a psychiatric module. It is, therefore, written at a depth relevant to this purpose. It will also prove useful to anyone who only has a brief period of time in which to gain insight into psychiatric nursing. It would be useful to students of physiotherapy and occupational therapy who work from time to time with psychiatric patients and to family planning nurses, midwives and community nurses who encounter people with mental health problems during the course of their daily work. That much-neglected group, the nursing auxillary or aide working in psychiatry, will find that it gives an insight into the theory behind the practice.

The reader is helped to recognize the problems, their causes and consequences and to identify ways of helping the person experiencing them, both in the institutional setting and community work. There are many competencies that are equally useful to general and psychiatric nurses wherever they happen to be caring for clients. The workbook can be used by the individual but can also be put to good use in group work, particularly if an experienced facilitator is present.

No particular model of nursing has been used and each chapter is approached in a different way. This is partly because there is no one way which is most appropriate and, if one specific model is used in a text of this kind, the learner is likely to find the transition to whatever model is being used within her place of work a more difficult one. My second reason is a more selfish one in that I myself become bored quite easily when reading textbooks unless there is variety in the presentation, just as learners will become bored if a tutor adopts the same method of teaching during each session of the school block. The exercises, none of which should take more than 30 minutes, form an integral part of the work. References and further reading lists are supplied for those who wish to follow up specific topics.

So often the problems of the psychiatric patient have been separated from those of the general patient. This is an artificial division since aggression, alcohol abuse and parasuicide are met with in the general setting very frequently. The person being nursed on a surgical ward following amputation may be just as depressed as the elderly lady confined to her home or the overdosed patient admitted to psychiatry.

During the past nine years I have taught general nursing students on their psychiatric modules and found that many of them look upon the experience with trepidation. By demystifying psychiatry and helping these nurses to see that the most frightening thing about psychiatric patients is their label, they can be encouraged to develop skills which can be transferred to any care setting in which they later find themselves. The simplicity of this book in no way denigrates the intelligence or motivation of this group of learners — it simply recognizes that they are bombarded with a huge amount and variety of information during their training and anything which gives just enough information must be a welcome break.

WENDY NGANASURIAN
1988

Introduction: Making the Most of your Time during the Mental Health Module

During your time as a student nurse you will spend a short period working in the mental health field, the aim of this module of experience being to introduce you to the range of facilities for, and help available to, people with mental health problems. You should also have the opportunity to work with people who suffer from mental illness, either in the acute stages of their illness or perhaps in a continuing care environment if the disorder becomes chronic. The allocation will probably provide the opportunity for you to develop some of the skills which you have used when working within the general nursing setting and to introduce some new aspects of these skills. The kinds of skill which you may have the opportunity to develop include those now to be described.

SKILLS IN DEVELOPING RELATIONSHIPS WITH CLIENTS/PATIENTS

Developing relationships is a very difficult task if the relationships are to have meaning and be therapeutic. Developing relationships involves using appropriate verbal and non-verbal communication in order to be approachable, recognizing the barriers to good relationships, and setting appropriate boundaries. Many nurses working in the psychiatric setting do not wear uniform and this in itself can be an influencing factor in relationships. It may foster a more personal approach and out of uniform you may find that you are less authoritative; but you are also individuals and some of you may feel, for a time, that you lack the protection of a uniform.

EXERCISE 1

Make a list of the advantages and disadvantages of wearing uniform in both the general and the psychiatric settings.

General setting

Advantages of wearing own clothing   *Advantages of wearing uniform*

Psychiatric setting

See if, at the end of your experience in the mental health module, you still feel the same.

SKILLS IN USING
COMMUNICATION THERAPEUTICALLY

It is interesting to see how freely some people can initiate a conversation with a stranger at a social level. For some people this is a skill that needs a lot of work, sometimes because, in psychiatry, people have preconceived ideas about what they should and should not say and may wonder what kind of odd reactions they will get from the patient. You will have the opportunity to initiate conversations related to people's problems, to listen to and encourage very distressed people, and to devise strategies for overcoming communication barriers. Sometimes, patients will not communicate verbally and this is an opportunity to develop the skill of 'reading' a person through their non-verbal communications.

EXERCISE 2

List ten reasons why someone might give a deep, long sigh.
1
2
3
4
5
6
7
8
9
10

SKILLS IN REDUCING ANXIETY

It is important to be able to act in a manner which is unlikely to create or increase anxiety in those around you. Nurses are always looked to in times of crisis because we are supposed to be able to stay calm when all others are losing their heads. You will be able to devise strategies to reduce anxiety in patients and these will stand you in good stead when you return to the general areas.

EXERCISE 3

On the 1–10 scales provided below (1 = low; 10 = high) rate how anxious you were when you started your last three allocations (or jobs if you have not had allocations) and rate how anxious you are now about starting in the psychiatric field.

Allocation 1

1(low)   2   3   4   5   6   7   8   9   10

Allocation 2

1   2   3   4   5   6   7   8   9   10

Allocation 3

1   2   3   4   5   6   7   8   9   10

Psychiatric allocation

1   2   3   4   5   6   7   8   9   10

Which was the highest in rating? Try to identify five or more reasons for your anxiety.

SKILLS IN REDUCING THE RISK OF SUICIDE

You will probably be made acutely aware of all the potential dangers since there are often people who may try to end their lives in a psychiatric unit or hospital. You will be asked to observe people both unobtrusively and closely, as the need dictates. Sometimes the word 'specialing' is used, describing the role of a nurse who has been allocated to stay with one particular patient and not leave his side. If you are allocated this role then it may be very stressful and you should discuss your feelings with the trained staff. It is a useful opportunity for you to spend time in a one-to-one interaction with someone who is distressed and it is very rewarding when, after recovery from the suicidal phase, a patient thanks you for the time and effort, kindness and consideration which you gave to him when he was feeling very low. There is nothing to be ashamed of in worrying over the responsibility that you feel has been put upon you, and admitting this is unlikely to be frowned upon.

SKILLS IN ADAPTING TO A DIFFERENT ENVIRONMENT AND TO DIFFERENT PATIENTS' NEEDS

The pace may be different, the routine different, the way people talk to each other, and so on. Patients probably do not need so much physical care and they may be more inclined to argue with you or ask for reasons and explanations. It is a skill to be able to change your own way of behaving as the environment demands. This is particularly true when you go out and visit people in their own homes or when engaged in social and recreational activities with patients outside the hospital's confines.

SKILLS IN CLARIFYING AND REINFORCING REALITY

You will possibly have the chance to use reality orientation during your module and you will certainly be dealing with patients who are confused, be it as a result of alcohol or drug abuse, dementia or head injury. There are many confused patients in geriatric wards, medical and surgical wards and even orthopaedic wards, and your skills can be transferred to these settings.

SKILLS IN REDUCING THE LIKELIHOOD OF AGGRESSION AND MANAGING AGGRESSIVE INCIDENTS

In contrast to what the public believes, very little physical aggression takes place in the psychiatric setting and it is more likely to occur in a geriatric ward or in the accident and emergency department than in a psychiatric ward. This may be because people develop the skill of recognizing when someone is tense or when an aggressive incident is likely to occur and take steps to alter the situation or intervene in some way. If an aggressive incident should occur, it is to be hoped that you will see the benefit of teamwork in dealing with it and you should pay particular attention to the way in which other patients in the ward are helped to deal with their feelings during and after such an incident.

SKILLS IN MOTIVATING CLIENTS/PATIENTS AND ACHIEVING A GREATER DEGREE OF COMPLIANCE

You will have ample opportunity to recognize what motivates people and implement these strategies. Encouraging compliance is a difficult skill to develop since each individual responds in a different way to requests, instructions, rewards, and so on. Nurses often complain that a patient will not comply with his diet or with his treatment plan or will not even remain in bed. You should use this opportunity to try to understand why people do not comply, and devise strategies for increasing the likelihood of compliance.

EXERCISE 4

If I asked you to stay in tonight and write the word 'house' as many times as possible what could I do to increase the chances of you doing it? Try to think about the environment you would be doing it in, relationships, rewards or incentives, reasons, outcomes, etc.

1
2
3
4
5
6
7
8
9
10

Could you apply any of these to a patient who would not comply with your request that he should try to walk for a little while each day?

SKILLS IN HELPING INDIVIDUALS TO MODIFY THEIR BEHAVIOUR

Behaviour modification is related to motivation, which we discussed in the previous section, but you will have the chance to identify, with the help of trained staff, inappropriate or self-defeating behaviour by various patients and to devise strategies to reduce or eliminate these behaviour patterns. This may occur while you are nursing a patient with anorexia or someone with an alcohol problem or a phobia. For instance, teaching someone to relax is a way of modifying his behaviour and can be used to great advantage in the general setting, particularly with a patient who is tense at night.

You will have plenty of opportunity to work on other skills such as self-awareness, assertiveness and the use of initiative. It is important that you should talk about your progress—it may take you a couple of weeks or more to settle into a different environment—but the mental health module can become an important part of a general nurse's training and—who knows—you may even find that you would like to undertake a psychiatric training course later on which will give you a much greater insight into all the things you have only touched on during the module.

It is the purpose of this book to give you an insight mainly into the theoretical aspects of mental health care, as I feel that learning the skills outlined above is best carried out in your clinical placements. However, there are numerous books that give good coverage of these skills if you are interested and wish to learn more about them; some of these books are listed in the further reading list which follows.

FURTHER READING

Longhorn, E. (1984) *Psychiatric Care and Conditions*. Chichester: John Wiley & Sons.
Martin, P. (1983) *Care of the Mentally Ill*. London: Macmillan.
Mitchell, R. (1986) *Essential Psychiatric Nursing*. Edinburgh: Churchill Livingstone.
Ward, M. (1986) *Learning to Care on the Psychiatric Ward*. London: Hodder & Stoughton.

Chapter 1

Mental Health Problems:
What is Mental Illness?

I was surprised one day by a telephone call from a friend.

'I've had a nervous breakdown,' she said. 'Oh I'm so sorry,' I replied, 'what happened?'

'Well,' she continued, 'I didn't know I'd had it until I read this book that someone gave me. You see, I thought a nervous breakdown was when you threw things around and went berserk but it isn't and I had just what they described.'

'Didn't you think there was anything wrong at the time?' I enquired.

'No, I just thought I was having one of my bad patches and John [her husband] says I've always been potty anyway.'

I think this illustrates quite nicely the question: 'What is mental illness?'

It is usually easy to identify when someone is physically ill. In fact, it is usually the individual himself who makes the initial global diagnosis of 'ill'. Physical illness produces a distortion of functioning in some way, a diagnosis can usually be made and a course of treatment commenced. If, for example, one has a cough it is labelled as an 'illness' if it is unpleasant and/or persistent. After self-medication has failed to relieve it, the sufferer goes to a doctor who probably makes a routine examination, labels the illness and prescribes something he believes will relieve it. If the sufferer wishes to confirm the diagnosis he can go to several other physicians who will most likely undertake a very similar examination and probably make the same diagnosis and prescribe the same treatment.

The process associated with mental health problems is not as clear-cut. It may be that the individual will himself recognize that he has a problem but it is sometimes someone else who will tell him that he needs help. We say that the patient has no insight if he cannot recognize his own disordered state. This means initially that the label of 'mental illness' may be applied by a layman who may use the term very loosely. It may simply mean that the individual labelled is doing something which the other person would not himself do or in some way does not conform to what the majority of people known to that person would do.

It is accepted that at certain times a person may progress along the continuum which represents at one end sanity, and at the other end illness. For example, a bereaved person is felt to be justified in his depression until someone comes along and says: 'I didn't react like that when I was bereaved', or 'It's gone on for too long—you ought to get some pills to help you cope.' The anxious person is justified in being anxious if an examination is coming up, but how much anxiety is normal? There is nothing wrong with checking that you have locked your front door once because 'everybody does it', but is it a sign of ill-health to check it twice or perhaps three or four times? What about the phobic who never uses a lift because he was once trapped in one? Is it rational behaviour never to use a lift again or should he seek help with the problem? So it remains that the layman continues to define mental ill-health in relation to the circumstances, his own mental state and that of the majority of the people he knows.

In distinguishing normal from the abnormal we have to ask what is meant by 'normal'. My *Pocket Oxford Dictionary* says it is 'the mean of the observed quantities'. It defines 'mean' as 'halfway between the highest and the lowest'. So if we look at the human race in those terms (for simplicity we confine our studies to the human race within England at the moment) we would have to establish who thinks what, how do they feel and what do they do. We could then identify what most of them thought, felt and did and there we have our mean. For example:

10 people say 'A'	100 people say 'B'	10 people say 'C'

Does this mean that the ten at either end are abnormal or are they just different? One hopes that the layman would say they were just different. If we were in a country that practised political control through psychiatry we could say that if ten people believe our system to be wrong but 100 believed it to be right then the ten are deluded (the term for a false belief). Treatment might be needed to correct their delusion! Even if we added to the above example a single person who says 'X' can we be so sure that he is ill or could it be that he sees things more clearly: perhaps he is right, or just different. If he is lucky enough to be rich we might even call him eccentric rather than mad.

Cochrane & Sobel (1980) defined mental illness as a 'valuable adaptive reaction that is resorted to when other forms of adaptation are not available or have been tried and felt to have failed'; therefore, mental illness is not an illness but a way of coping. Some people, especially some of those with medical qualifications, may look upon problems of living as illnesses or diseases which are treatable with drugs as the primary therapeutic agent. However, it is becoming more acceptable to look at mental health problems as ways of reacting to certain situations and the 'mentally ill' as people who have problems with living. Rosenham (1975) showed that it was very difficult for the psychiatric services to differentiate between health and ill-health in the mental field (see Chapter 2) but if you do get agreement between two psychiatrists (the experts) over whether the individual is ill or not then you are unlikely to get agreement over the specific diagnosis. It is interesting to listen to consultants debating whether a patient is schizophrenic, manic-depressive or psychopathic, each one putting forward a good case for why he is right.

Let us look at a surgical example. Imagine that your leg has been amputated. It would seem to be inappropriate if you were happy about the situation. Of course, if the amputation was to have beneficial effects then to be happy *would* be appropriate. For example, it might be necessary in order to prolong your life or to enable you to walk again once a prosthesis had been fitted. It might be that you think there could be advantages to living in a wheelchair because someone close to you would be less likely to leave you now you are dependent on them, or perhaps it's a way of getting out of work or gaining financial compensation. We find it hard to imagine that anything could compensate for a leg being amputated and so we judge the happiness according to what we think we would feel or what we believe the majority of people would feel. If this same amputation resulted in depression that also seems to be reasonable, but if the depressed person refuses to eat, cannot sleep, and does not want to speak then that depression becomes an illness—or does it?

By now you are probably thinking, 'Oh dear, why didn't I just stick to something nice and simple with everything black and white and nicely fitting into neat slots?' Psychiatry is not like that and this may partly explain why early days during a psychiatric module can be very confusing. Horses may be quite comfortable in blinkers and people can be comfortable if they only look straight ahead and never to the sides.

If we take a look at depression it may help to illustrate why only a few people actually end up in hospital labelled as ill when huge numbers of people understand the symptoms.

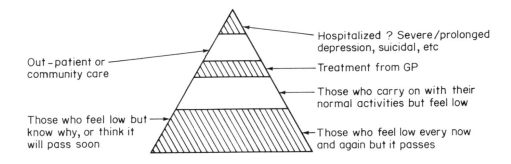

The World Health Organization identifies and names mental illnesses according to the following classification (only the most commonly encountered disorders are included):

Psychoses	*Neuroses*
(a) Functional psychoses	Anxiety state
Schizophrenia	Phobia
Manic-depressive psychosis	Obsessive–compulsive state
(i) manic type	Hysterical neurosis
(ii) depressive type	
(iii) cyclical type	*Personality disorders*
Paranoid illnesses	Psychopathy (sociopathy)
(b) Organic psychoses	
Acute brain syndrome (delirium or confusional state)	*Alcohol and drug dependence*
Chronic brain syndrome (dementia)	
Psychosomatic disorders	*Psychosexual disorders*
Miscellaneous disorders	
Anorexia nervosa	
Bulimia nervosa	

One way of looking at mental health problems is to use what the individual tells us are his problems and the consequences of these. Mental health problems rarely affect the individual alone. Members of the systems in which he functions are involved. The trend is now towards giving help with mental health problems in the community rather than removing the sufferer from his family and normal surroundings. If we get away from the 'illness model' we may find that one day we will not need a place called a hospital, staffed with people called doctors and nurses, in order to help people who have problems with living.

EXERCISE 1

How do you rate yourself in the mental health stakes. Here are twenty positive health statements: acknowledge each one by using the grading system on the right of the page and placing a tick in the appropriate column. A tick in column X means that the statement applies fully to you, and one in column Y means that the statement is not characteristic of you.

If the statement applies more often than not, tick the 'tendency to X' column and if it does not apply to you for most of the time tick the 'tendency to Y' column. It is important that you try to be ruthlessly honest with yourself—after all, you do not have to show your answers to anyone else!

	Grading			
	X	Tendency to X	Tendency to Y	Y
1. I take a well-balanced diet and sufficient fluids to maintain normal weight and fluid/electrolyte balance				
2. I obtain sufficient rest and sleep to meet my body's physiological requirements and to feel refreshed				
3. I take enough exercise to prevent the complications of inactivity				
4. I breathe adequately to meet my body's respiratory requirements				
5. I eliminate waste from my body comfortably				
6. I achieve a state of pain-free physiological homeostasis				
7. I appreciate my personal strengths and weaknesses realistically whilst maintaining an overall positive self-image				
8. I achieve success and satisfaction in personal relationships, work and social activities				
9. I divide my time in such a way as to carry out all that is needed without undue pressure				
10. I make realistic interpretations based on observations and information that I receive				
11. I minimize danger to myself and others				

continued on next page

continued

	Grading			
	X	Tendency to X	Tendency to Y	Y
12. I obtain pleasure in expressing thoughts and feelings in a manner which does not cause offence to others				
13. I find satisfaction through recreational/relaxational activities				
14. I maintain an adequate and acceptable roof over my head				
15. I look positively towards my future and am motivated to continue living				
16. I set realistic goals and make appropriate decisions independently				
17. I look after myself without having to rely on others to meet my needs				
18. I satisfy my sexual needs within my cultural boundaries				
19. I practise my own philosophy of life or religion to my own satisfaction and without causing offence or nuisance to others				
20. I function in the company of others in such a way as to satisfy myself and not unduly interfere with the functioning of others				

Having answered the statements, look to see if you have any ticks in the Y columns. If you have can you identify what it is that prevents you from answering positively and could you change it?

REFERENCES

Cochrane, R. & Sobel, M. (1980) Life stresses and psychological consequences. In *The Social Psychology of Psychological Problems*. Chichester: John Wiley & Sons.

Rosenhan, D. (1975) On being sane in insane places. *Science*, **179**, 250–258.

FURTHER READING

Barton, P. *et al.* (1985) *The Politics of Mental Health*. London: Macmillan.

Barton P. (1986) *Patient Assessment in Psychiatric Nursing*. London: Croom Helm.

Cox, L. (ed.) (1986) *Transcultural Psychiatry*. London: Croom Helm.

Chapter 2

Causes and Consequences of Mental Ill-health

EXERCISE 1

Make a list of everything which you would classify as being stressful that has happened to you during the preceding year. When you have done this try to establish what it was about each of these things that was stressful and what emotions accompanied them. For example, you might have attended a family wedding and found it stressful, perhaps because you had difficulty in getting the time off, or you were in a rush on the day trying to have your hair done, or you were a bridesmaid and knew that all eyes would be on you at times, and so on. The emotions that you identify may include anxiety, happiness or excitement.

Having completed this part of the exercise, now consider if there is anything that you might have done which could have made these events less stressful.

WHAT CAUSES MENTAL ILL-HEALTH?

Life events and environmental factors	Genetic factors
Upbringing	Biochemical factors
Personality and self-image factors	Cerebral pathology

Genetic Factors

Some psychiatric disorders are known to be inherited. For example, Huntington's chorea is passed on through a dominant gene on an autosomal chromosome: this means that because the gene is dominant, every child of an affected parent stands a 50:50 chance of inheriting the disorder. Since it is on an autosomal chromosome, either sex is equally likely to be affected and it does not actually 'skip' a generation, although a parent may die of some other cause before the symptoms of Huntington's chorea become apparent.

With some disorders a link has been established which suggests a genetic cause. For example, researchers have studied twins who were adopted away from alcoholic parents (Goodwin 1973) and found a high rate of alcoholism even though there was no environmental influence with the adoptive parents, as there would have been if the children had stayed with their alcoholic parents. The concordance rate in most twin studies is higher when monozygotic twins are compared with dizygotic twins since the former share exactly the same genetic makeup, coming from the same egg. This is also true when studying schizophrenia (Gottesman & Shields 1973). Studies have also shown a familial link for some types of affective disorders (Kolb 1977).

Biochemistry

Excess of the neurotransmitter dopamine has been suggested as a cause of schizophrenia, low levels of noradrenaline for depression, high levels of serotonin for anxiety, and low levels of acetylcholine for Alzheimer's disease.

Cerebral Pathology

Toxins, trauma, tumours, infections, including a slow virus, hypoxia and raised aluminium levels may all produce temporary or permanent pathological changes in the brain cells. In dementia, brain cells die at an increased rate. Research is going on into the possibility of an autoimmune process whereby for some reason certain people develop antibodies which destroy their brain cells.

Personality and Self-image Factors

Our personality is the product of our inheritance, our upbringing and our experiences. Some people are more prone to mental illness because their personality makes them vulnerable. For example, it may be that some people find any pressure put on them intolerable and respond by withdrawing. Others cannot see solutions to problems or tolerate any frustration, and resort to the abuse of alcohol and drugs. For many people guilt features greatly in their personality while others are continually suspicious of people's motives. Some people never feel right about themselves and become hypercritical, isolated and unhappy.

Seligman (1975) developed the theory of 'learned helplessness' through experiments on dogs. According to his theory some people feel that they have little or no control over their lives and need help from others in order to function. Beck (1979) believes that the way some people think causes them to become depressed, always extracting and maximizing the negative happenings in their lives.

People sometimes relate to a role. For example, a woman might identify herself and her self-worth only in relation to others. Being a wife or mother may be so important to her that when these roles disappear she feels lost. If a woman sees herself as no longer feminine, attractive or desirable, or a man feels he is about as 'macho' as a doormouse, the self-image becomes damaged and depression may follow. Pitt (1980) describes the 'panic over unrealized ambitions, the awful feeling that life is unlikely to alter much, the trapped sense of "this is it"' which may accompany middle age.

Upbringing

Parents, or parent substitutes, have a tremendous responsibility if their offspring are to grow up well-balanced. Imagine, for example, never being able to please one's parents, always being compared unfavourably with a preferred sibling or being separated from a parent early in life. Both Bowlby (1973) and Munro (1969) looked at the significance of this latter occurrence and related it to the development of depression and suicide in later life. Being given 'double-bind' communications (Bateson *et al.* 1956)—that is, two contradictory messages being sent at once—has been associated with the development of schizophrenia. An example is the parent saying 'That's OK, you do as you please, don't worry about me', while at the same time looking angry or hurt. Parents may make a scapegoat of a child and blame him for anything that is wrong within the family. Laing (1967) believes that the symptoms we call schizophrenia may simply be a very sensible way of living within an intolerable family situation.

A child might witness the obsessional routines of a parent and model himself on this behaviour. He might witness, or be the victim of, physical abuse and this may engender guilt, fear or even mimicry. If a child never receives love he may be unable to give love.

Life Events and Environmental Factors

Life is full of stress. Charles Spielberger, in *Understanding Stress and Anxiety* (1979), defines stress as referring to 'both the circumstances that place physical or psychological demands on an individual and the emotional reactions experienced in these situations'. The stresses we face are often associated with the 'not enoughs' or the 'too much' factors. The 'not enoughs' include money, time, love, work, and the 'too much' group includes work, status, love, noise and time.

Being married seems to cause problems particularly for women, since figures suggest that more married women than single women are hospitalized for psychiatric disorders. However, more single men than married men are hospitalized. Having a baby may be stressful enough to produce the first episode of mental illness. Loss is an extremely significant life event. The loss may be through death, or simply through the ending of a relationship, but it may also be a role that ends, such as loss of work through illness, retirement or redundancy.

There are significant social class differences when looking at the epidemiology of mental disorder and, generally speaking, the lower the class the higher the rate of illness. This area can be studied in depth since it brings in such factors as the doctor's willingness to diagnose a psychotic or other serious condition in someone of his own social class and the compatibility of verbal and non-verbal communication between the carers and the identified patient. Wardle (1967) suggests that if the patient cannot make himself clear to us he is more likely to be called psychotic or perhaps we just do not really bother to listen to him if he is in a lower social class. Certainly, doctors spend less time with lower social class clients during interviews (Cartwright & O'Brien 1976). Cultural differences are important since there appears to be a higher rate of mental disorder in ethnic minority groups. Once all kinds of adjustment have been made to these figures using age, sex, etc., as Cochrane did (1977), the rates are not really that high.

CONSEQUENCES OF MENTAL ILL-HEALTH

An important consequence of mental illness is the very label itself. A label is a way of categorizing or describing something or someone. Szasz (1982) maintains that 'a label prescribes, not describes': in other words, it is a self-fulfilling prophecy (the individual will take on the behaviour appropriate to that role) and the label tells others what to look for and determines what they will see.

This is well illustrated by Rosenhan (1973) who arranged for mentally healthy individuals to fake mental illness in order to be admitted to psychiatric hospitals. Once admitted they reverted to their normal behaviour and, of course, should have been released because their mental ill-health episode was obviously over: however, the last one to be released had spent 52 days in psychiatric care. Once the label is applied it is hard to disprove it. Laing (1967) suggests that if you are labelled insane and protest that you are not, that is evidence of your insanity and only when you show insight, i.e. admit to your 'illness', are you seen to be on the road to recovery since you now have insight, which is a good sign. Scheff (1975) maintains that if we accept a label and adopt the 'sick role' we are rewarded for it, but Doherty found (1975) that those who accepted their role recovered more slowly than those who fought against it. This label is stigmatizing and affects the individual's chances of work; it affects the way people interact with him, it diminishes his credibility, and it will be used repeatedly throughout the individual's life, even after recovery. Society only sympathsizes with those who did not bring about their own illness through their behaviour. Many mental disorders do not appear to fit this criterion and, therefore, the sympathy accorded to the sick does not follow a diagnosis of mental illness in many cases. Alcoholism, drug dependence and, in some instances, depression may be looked upon as being of one's own making.

As a consequence of mental illness we may be hospitalized, perhaps removing us from the causes of our problems or putting us into a situation where the problems are unlikely to recur. This may be comfortable, safe and secure, and as long as we can accept the loss of individuality or independence that may go with being hospitalized we may then recover enough to continue our lives, but only for as long as we can remain in the institution. When any changes threaten to occur, the individual may resist them: soon he would become 'streetwise' to the ways of the total institution, as described by Goffman in his book *Asylum*

(1968). People take on the norms which belong to the deviant subculture in which they currently reside.

Even after discharge it is possible to become stuck in the 'revolving door' when the periods of time outside hospital (supposedly periods of remission or recovery) get shorter and the in-patient periods get longer. The policy of closing large, traditional hospitals and developing community psychiatric facilities should go some way towards the prevention of institutionalization as we know it, with its isolation from the society surrounding the institution. Staying with one's problems in the community may be more beneficial if there are people there to help, and somewhere to go for a period of respite when necessary rather than escaping from them into an artificial environment.

The consequences of mental illness upon the carers may be that an unbearable burden is imposed on them. One only has to imagine what it must be like to live with someone who is profoundly depressed or paranoid to gain some appreciation of the problem. In *The 36-hour Day* (Mace & Rabin 1985) the kinds of problem faced by someone coping with a dementing relative come to light. For all families with a mentally-ill relative there are physical consequences such as the exhaustion arising from constant caring, washing and watching, the emotional consequences such as the guilt arising from one's feelings about the sick person and the social consequences of, for example, being unable or, if it is the breadwinner who is sick, not being able to afford to go out.

EXERCISE 2

> Imagine that you have been admitted to a psychiatric hospital or unit. Make a list on one side of a sheet of paper of all the things you think you could get to like about being in hospital, and on the other side all the things you would not like.

EXERCISE 3

> Imagine that you have just landed from Mars in the middle of a psychiatric institution. What behaviour would you have to adopt in order to blend in completely with the Earth people there, including how you should dress, walk, talk, etc? How close are the norms of this deviant subculture to those of society? In the hospital or psychiatric unit which you are working in what could be done in order to make the environment, and what goes on within it, more like what happens in the community outside?

SELF-EVALUATION

1 What causes Huntington's chorea?
2 What would be the chances of the child of an affected parent having the disorder?
3 What is meant by the term monozygotic?
4 Why is it important to study both dizygotic and monozygotic twins who were adopted away from ill parents?
5 What is a neurotransmitter? Name three.
6 What is a 'double-bind'?
7 What was found to have happened in the early life of many people who were profoundly depressed or suicidal?
8 Which social class is shown in epidemiological surveys to have the highest rates of psychiatric morbidity? How might this be explained in relation to the way the diagnosis is made?
9 What is meant by a 'self-fulfilling prophecy', and how does it apply in mental illness?
10 Identify three reasons why patients may get stuck in the 'revolving door'.

Answers will be found on p. 89.

REFERENCES

Bateson, G., Jackson, D., Haley, J. & Weakland, J. (1956) Towards a theory of schizophrenia. Behavioural Science, **1**, 251–264.
Beck, L. (1979) *Cognitive Theory of Depression*. New York: Guildford Press.
Birch, A. (1983) *What Chance do We Have*. MIND—National Association for Mental Health.
Bitt, B. (1980) *Mid-life Crises*. London: Sheldon Press.
Bowlby, J. (1973) *Separation, Attachment and Loss*, Vol 2. New York: Basic Books.
Cartwright, A. & O'Brien, M. (1976) Social class variations in health care in the nature of GP consultations. In Stacey, M. (ed.) *Sociology of the National Health Service*. Sociological Review Monograph No. 22: Wood Mitchell, 77–98.
Cochrane, R. (1977) Psychological and behaviour disturbances in West Indians and Pakistanis in Britain: a comparison of rates among children and adults. *British Journal of Psychiatry*, **134**, 201–210.
Doherty, E. (1975) Labelling effects in psychiatric hospitalization. *Archives of General Psychiatry*, **32**, 562–572.
Fagin, L. & Little, M. (1984) *The Forsaken Families*. Harmondsworth: Pelican Books.
Goffman, E. (1961) *Asylums*. Harmondsworth: Penguin Books.
Goffman, E. (1968) *Stigma: Notes on the Management of Spoiled Identity*. Harmondsworth: Penguin Books.
Gotesman, I. & Shields, J. (1972) *Schizophrenia and Genetics. A Twin Study Vantage Point*. New York: Academic Press.
Gotesman, I. & Shields, J. (1973) Genetic theorising and schizophrenia. *British Journal of Psychiatry*, **122**, 13–30.
Hase, S. & Douglas, A. (1986) *Human Dynamics and Nursing*. Edinburgh: Churchill Livingstone.
Hollingshead, A. & Redlich, F. (1958) *Social Class and Mental Illness*. New York: John Wiley & Sons.
Laing, R. D. (1967) *The Politics of Experience*. London: Pantheon Press.

Laing, R. D. & Esterson, A. (1964) *Sanity, Madness and the Family*. Harmondsworth: Penguin Books.
Lodge, B. (1981) *Coping with Caring*. London: MIND—National Association for Mental Health.
Mace, N. & Rabins, P. (1985) *The 36-hour Day*. London: Age Concern.
Munro, A. (1969) Parent/child separation. *Archives of General Psychiatry*, **20**, 598–604.
Rosenhan, D. (1975) On being sane in insane places. *Science*, **179**, 250–258.
Scheff, T. (ed.) (1975) *Labelling Madness*. New York: Prentice-Hall.
Seligman, M. (1975) *Helplessness*. London: W. H. Freeman.
Szasz, T. (1982) *The Myth of Mental Illness*. St Albans: Paladin Books.
Wardle, C. (1967) Social factors in the major functional psychoses. In Welford, A. T., Argyle, M., Glass,
     D. & Morris, J. (eds) *Society: Problems and Methods of Study*. London: Routledge & Kegan Paul, 19.

FURTHER READING

Cochrane, R. (1983) *The Social Stress of Mental Illness*. Colchester: Longman.
Mangen, S. (1982) *Sociology and Mental Health*. Edinburgh: Churchill Livingstone.
Scheff, T. (ed.) (1967) *Mental Illness and Social Processes*. New York: Harper & Row.
Spielberger, C. (1979) *Understanding Stress and Anxiety*. New York: Harper & Row.

Chapter 3

Legal Aspects of Psychiatric Care

The Mental Health Act 1983 is a large and complicated legal document. It is important for psychiatric nurses to understand the Act in depth and there is usually someone on the administration staff who deals with all queries which cannot be dealt with at ward level. Legal advice can always be sought and there are regular visits from the Mental Health Act Commission who monitor the interpretation and implementation of the Act in each hospital or psychiatric department. For the purpose of this book it is sufficient for us to have a somewhat simplified look at the Act in order to gain a basic understanding of the way in which it protects patients, the public and staff.

The most usual route to psychiatric care is when the patient or his family goes to their *general practitioner* complaining of, or showing signs of, mental illness. The general practitioner may treat them himself or refer them to a psychiatrist.

The *psychiatrist* sees them on a *domicillary visit* or in the *outpatient department* either by appointment or as an emergency.

Following assessment the psychiatrist will decide which *care option* he favours. These are (a) continue with outpatient appointments; (b) care within the community including attendance at a day hospital or with community psychiatric nurse follow-up; (c) inpatient care.

If he considers the patient to be in need of *inpatient care* he will ask if the patient is *willing* to come in.

continued on next page

---

continued

If the patient is willing he will be admitted as an *informal patient*. There may be a waiting-list if it is not urgent.

↓

If he considers the patient needs *in-patient care* but the patient is *not willing* to agree to this he has to decide if the patient is either a *danger to himself or to others*. If the answer is 'yes' then he has the power to admit the patient *compulsorily* by placing him/her on a section of the *Mental Health Act* 1983.

↓

To place anyone on a section of this Act a strict procedure has to be followed. For some sections, e.g. Section 4, it is necessary to obtain a signature on the application from either the *nearest relative* of the patient or a *specially approved social worker*, plus a *medical recommendation* supporting their application. This can be done by the GP because he knows the patient better than any other doctor. Section 4 lasts for 72 hours but if the patient is to be put on one of the longer sections, e.g. Section 2 (28 days) or Section 3 (6 months and renewable), two doctors are required to support the application. One of these doctors should know the patient and one should have special knowledge of psychiatry.

↓

If admitted *informally* the patient has the right *to discharge himself* and *to refuse treatment*. Treatment can only be given to him against his wishes if, for example, he is acting in a way which constitutes a danger or is disruptive to treatment, by using common law principles which apply throughout medicine in general. This last statement also applies to patients on short duration sections, i.e. those lasting for 72 hours or less.

↓

If *compulsorily detained* (on Section 2 or 3 or certain court orders but NOT on short-duration sections), the patient *must* accept certain treatments. However, *his consent is always needed* before hormone implants or psychosurgery can be carried out. He also has the right to refuse to have electro-convulsive therapy and, likewise, he can refuse to accept drug treatments once he has been receiving them for a three-month period. If, however, his medical officer considers it to be essential that he should have ECT, or that he should continue to receive drugs, a *second medical opinion* may be sought from the Mental Health Act Commission and if they agree to the necessity the treatments will be administered against the patient's wishes. Certain treatments also may be given in emergency and the need for consent may be waived. For more details, see sections 57, 58 and 62 of the Act.

continued on next page

continued

As a *compulsorily detained* patient he is not allowed to leave without permission and can be *brought back by the police* if he does so.

When the period for which he is *detained compulsorily* comes to an end the patient may become *informal*, assuming that he is not yet ready for discharge, or *another section* may be applied or his *existing section renewed*, depending on the section under which he was detained.

Any patient, whether informal or compulsorily detained, must be *informed of his rights*. This is usually done on admission and again when the patient is at his most lucid and able to comprehend the information more fully. A patient on the longer-duration sections has the *right to appeal* to the Mental Health Review Tribunal who may, after considering the individual case, order the patient's release from section.

Psychiatric patients are protected by law from *physical and sexual abuse by staff* and from *financial exploitation*. If they have property or money it may be handled by the *Court of Protection* which acts in their best interests until they are able to resume control. A patient may make *a will* if his doctor considers him to be of sound testamentary capacity.

SELF-EVALUATION

1 Under what circumstances may a patient come into hospital as an informal patient?
2 Can any form of treatment be given to an informal patient against his wishes if it is not an emergency?
3 Which treatments may not be given to any patient who is unwilling to have them?
4 Can you give drugs to a patient who is detained on section 3?
5 Which treatments can be given to a patient who is on section 3, even if he or she is unwilling to have them, if a second medical opinion is in agreement with the patient's doctor about the necessity for such treatments?
6 Can the police bring back a patient who is informal and has left the hospital without permission?
7 What is the name of the body to which a compulsorily detained patient may appeal against detention on a section of the Act?
8 What is the name of the body which visits hospitals to monitor the functioning and application of the Act?

continued on next page

continued

---

9 Who would have to sign the section papers if a person was being placed on section 2 of the Act?

10 Although this has not been mentioned, what do you think would happen if an informally-detained patient decided to discharge himself but the staff considered that he was a danger to himself or to others?

Answers will be found on p. 89.

FURTHER READING

Campbell, A. (1987) Forensic psychiatry and legal aspects of psychiatry. *Medicine International*, July, 190.

Chapter 4

Different Ways of Showing Anxiety

ANXIETY STATE

Anxiety may arise as a result of a stressful situation which we are aware of but sometimes we may be unaware of its cause: in other words, the origins of our anxiety may be conscious or unconscious. For example, an examination is generally seen as being a stressful event and we would be aware of the reason for our feelings of anxiety. However, this is not the case in the following example:

> A man admitted to the psychiatric unit knew of no reason for the sudden onset of his anxiety state. He presented with all the features of this condition but no apparent cause for it. His history revealed that some five years previously he had been working on a government contract in Africa when there had been a military coup and a sudden change of government. He and the other expatriates had been advised to leave very quickly. There had been no time to think or worry, just pack and get out. The situation was dangerous and one of his colleagues (although he hardly knew him) was killed. He had returned to England and worked as a civil engineer for over four years before the symptoms developed. Once he was able to relive his African experiences and face up to how he had felt at the time he could then recognize the origins of his anxiety.

Some people suffer from chronic anxiety, which remains with them despite treatment. For some there is an identifiable starting point (as in the patient who relates her first episode of anxiety to just after the birth of her first child), but for others there is no event that they can relate it to, the cause perhaps being deeply buried in the unconscious mind. Some people suffer from anxiety only in specific situations, and this is referred to as *phobia*. Someone might, for example, only be anxious or even panic-stricken near a dog or when he has to travel in a train.

It is easy to grasp the physical, psychological and behavioural changes seen in an anxiety state if we can understand the mechanism of stress.

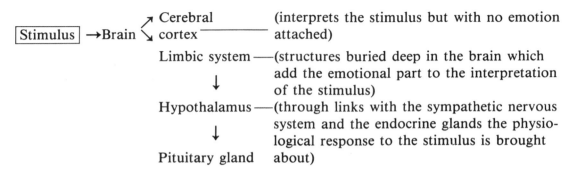

23

Physical changes	*Psychological and behavioural changes*
Dilated pupils, sweating, tremor, restlessness, tachycardia, increased respirations, dry mouth, adrenaline and glucose mobilized.	Inability to concentrate or settle, irritability, easily moved to tears, indecisive, feelings of dread. Pacing, fidgeting, worry over physical symptoms.

HYSTERICAL NEUROSIS

Sometimes as a result of intolerable stress, anxiety may not reveal itself as such: instead, it is revealed in the development of symptoms of physical or mental illness. These symptoms are real to the sufferer although there is no demonstrable pathology. In other words, the mind causes an arm to become paralysed or the individual to lose his memory but there is, of course, no nerve or muscle damage, nor brain damage, and no disease process or trauma to account for this.

> Amanda, a pretty 22-year-old girl, who had been engaged to Tony for two years, was admitted to a general hospital. They were due to marry soon after her return from university. As the wedding date approached she began to have doubts about the decision but did not want to hurt Tony, nor did she want to risk losing him completely. She felt unable to discuss this with him or anyone else. Three weeks before her wedding she developed paralysis of both legs and was admitted to hospital. She was in no way malingering (consciously pretending or faking illness): she could not walk. This served a useful purpose in that it relieved her anxiety about the wedding and the decision to spend her life with Tony but it also had certain rewards (called secondary gains) attached to it. For example, people, especially her parents, were not cross with her even though much money had already been spent on the wedding. In fact everyone, including Tony, was attentive and loving towards her. The symbolism is easy to see — she could not walk up the aisle.

Hysterical conversion reactions, as these physical manifestations are called, may be looked upon as a flight from intolerable stress into illness. Conversion is one of the mental defence mechanisms which we all use to help us to cope with situations where our self-image, and the picture of ourselves we offer to others, is threatened. We do not consciously choose which of the many mental defence mechanisms we use. Hysterical conversion may take the form of paralysis, blindness, deafness, inability to speak, fits or a portrayal of mental illness (pseudodementia).

Sometimes the individual displays hysterical dissociative features. Dissociation is another mental defence mechanism, in which patients present with hysterical amnesia: they cannot remember who they are or how they got where they are.

> A man was taken to the psychiatric hospital after having been found sitting in a cemetery by the police. He told them that he did not know how he got there, what he was doing there or who he was. Within a few days his memory returned bit by bit and it transpired that his wife was leaving him and his business was collapsing. It was his way of getting a period of 'time out' so to speak — he did not have to think about the future because he did not know how to face it.

> In another instance, a father who had witnessed his two young children killed in a fire was admitted to a psychiatric ward. His wife was seriously ill in hospital. He could not remember anything about the fire or what happened afterwards, although he was present throughout.

Very rarely, dissociation takes the form of the person having two or more personalities which may be unaware of each other. The famous film *The Three Faces of Eve* is an example of a woman who had three distinctly different personalities and even had different handwriting and dresses for each one.

Dr Jekyll, and his alter ego Mr Hyde, is an example of a symbolic multiple personality, although initially he uses a drug to bring out the other personality.

There are two other hysterical reactions which a general nurse may encounter. One is Briquet's syndrome in which the patient presents with a long history of numerous physical complaints, all of which have no physical origin; the other is Münchausen's syndrome, or 'hospital addiction', in which a person obtains admission for investigation or operation on numerous occasions. In the latter, malingering is a more appropriate term because this patient will consciously fake the illness. However, such a person must be extremely disturbed psychologically to want to go through all that he endures in order to get the positive benefits of a caring environment, and he needs psychiatric help rather than derision.

OBSESSIVE–COMPULSIVE NEUROSIS

Anxiety may hide itself under ritualistic behaviour. After all, if you wash your hands fifty times a day there will be little time in which to concentrate on anything else but handwashing! The analytical view is that the obsessive–compulsive behaviour (obsessions being repetitive thoughts, and compulsions repeated acts) arises when unconscious and somewhat distasteful ideas creep up to consciousness in the mind. Therefore, if we have slightly 'dirty' or 'sinful' thoughts the way to stop them may be to control what we do, leaving no time for anything else. We might wash ourselves repeatedly, symbolically cleaning away our dirty thoughts. The behavioural school would say that we had learnt to carry out the behaviour at some time as a result of some experience, and as anxiety mounts we relieve it by performing the compulsions: this brings about temporary relief of the anxiety.

A 48-year-old female patient was the supervisor of a typing pool for a large city company. One night before going home she happened to look into a wastepaper basket and saw there an important document. She wondered how often this had happened without her knowledge and decided to check the bins. She looked at every piece of paper in every bin but found nothing. She repeated this behaviour for several days. Then one evening when she was just about to go home after her usual bin check she began to doubt her own thoroughness. In order to ensure that she had not missed something she repeated her check. From then on she began to check each bin twice automatically. This was sufficient for a while but soon she began to doubt even the second check. She tried to resist the urge to check a third time but the anxiety which resisting the urge produced was so great that she decided it was the lesser of two evils to make a third check. Soon she found that when she got home she was still totally obsessed with the doubt that she had not checked properly and sought help through her doctor.

Another female patient was admitted to the psychiatric unit having developed an obsessional fear that she would harm herself or someone else with knife. Her husband would lock all the knives in the garage when he left for work and this had gone on for months without either of them seeking help.

MEDICAL AND NURSING INTERVENTIONS FOR THE
RELIEF OF ANXIETY AND RELATED DISORDERS

Counselling Approach

The usual approach is to try, if possible, to identify the cause. Through counselling we look at the effect of the manifestations, be they of an hysterical or an obsessional nature. The individual is helped to express his anxieties in an acceptable verbal manner and to identify alternative coping strategies. Physical symptoms should be explained in a realistic manner.

Relationships

It is important to let the client know that he is accepted and valued and understood even though his behaviour may be seen by himself or others as being silly, 'over the top', and so on. The client is encouraged to develop a trusting relationship with staff in which he can be himself and express his true feelings without fear of rejection by any members of staff.

Medication

Some clients may be helped by prescribed anxiolytics such as diazepam. These should only be prescribed for a maximum of four months since they do not relieve anxiety after this period and physical dependence is a danger. Modified narcosis (sleep treatment) may be prescribed to relieve the exhaustion of anxiety, and drug-induced abreaction (releasing pent-up emotions and helping the client to talk by the use of intravenous drug administration) may be offered.

Behavioural Approach

Relaxation may be taught. The individual may be given a chart on which to keep a record of when his anxiety is greatest and what preceded the feelings. The client may be asked to produce some kind of hierarchy of situations in which he feels anxious. Response-limitation schemes may be introduced to reduce the amount of time spent in ritualistic or obsessional activity. All desirable behaviour should be rewarded with attention and undesirable elements of behaviour either ignored to minimize the effect they have or treated in a matter-of-fact way. For example, a patient with hysterical paralysis of an arm may be shown how best to get dressed and then left to get on with it. He may be encouraged to perform passive exercises using a statement like: 'Your mind will not let your arm work at the moment but when you *can* use it you won't be able to unless you have kept the muscle active.' If the client collapses to the floor or fits hysterically he is simply offered a hand to get up with no judgement passed but no reward offered either. The phobic may be asked to work through his fears, starting with the least frightening aspects and continuing through a hierarchy to the most frightening thing that he can imagine happening to him.

Diversional and Occupational Approaches

The individual may need to be diverted from thinking about his physical state or the obsessional activity that he wishes to carry out. If something can be found to interest him and give him the opportunity to express his feelings creatively, but without the stress of competition, this will help.

PHYSICAL CARE

Anxiety may interfere with eating and sleeping and with personal care. It is important that the client gets sufficient sleep and rest, even if drugs have to be resorted to, although relaxation training and other sleep-inducing techniques are preferable. If solid food is unattractive, fluid substitutes such as 'Build-Up' may be offered. The client should be encouraged to continue to attend to his personal hygiene and appearance and the relaxing effect of a warm bath emphasized, particularly before bed. Likewise, a short walk in the fresh air often helps one to relax and sleep later on.

EXERCISE 1

You may find it useful to study Chapter 12 before completing this exercise.

How might you deal with the following problems presented by a patient on a surgical ward?

1   A patient due for surgery later in the week is obviously anxious and very tense.
2   Following surgery, a patient constantly complains of various aches, pains, difficulty in walking and from time to time falls to the floor, especially when asked to walk. He has been examined thoroughly and there is no physical foundation for his symptoms.
3   A patient insists upon cleaning the bath with scouring powder for a full half-hour before she will get in it and again for half-an-hour when she gets out.

How might you deal with the following situation which occurs when you are working in the community?

Your patient will have to go into hospital soon for a relatively minor operation. However, she has told you that she is hospital-phobic and thinks it really will be impossible for her to have the operation even though she understands why it is necessary.

SELF-EVALUATION

1   What is meant by specific or situational anxiety?
2   Where would you find the limbic system and what is its function?
3   What effect would stimulation of the sympathetic nervous system have on the following organs?
     (a) heart
     (b) bronchioles
     (c) mouth
     (d) pupils
     (e) skin
     (f) bladder
4   What is a mental defence mechanism?
5   Give an example of a hysterical conversion reaction and explain why it may be described as symbolic.
6   What type of disorder is a multiple personality?
7   What is meant by Briquet's syndrome?
8   How do Briquet's syndrome and Munchausen's syndrome differ?
9   What is meant by 'response limitation'?
10   Mrs Chandler has not been out of the house for eight months. She becomes anxious to the point of panic when she leaves her home. She has a husband and two young children. (a) How may her problem have affected relationships and life within the family? (b) How might she be helped? (Use the information which has already been given concerning medical and nursing interventions.)

Answers will be found on p. 90.

FURTHER READING

Lyttle, J. (1986) *Mental Disorder: Its Care and Treatment*. Eastbourne: Baillière Tindall.
Ward, M. (1986) *Learning to Care on the Psychiatric Ward*. London: Hodder & Stoughton.
Whitehead, T. (1980) *Fears and Phobias*. Norwich: Fletcher & Sons.

Chapter 5

The Ups and Downs of Feelings

In this chapter we look at the problems which may cause one to feel very low and how feeling very low in turn causes problems. It is often a 'chicken and egg' situation — for example, is John Brown feeling low in mood because he has no friends and cannot mix well with people, or is it his low mood which results in his being unable to make friends and mix well? Whichever way round it is, we know that John Brown has a problem in making friends and mixing.

Feelings or emotions are sometimes referred to as 'affect' hence the term 'affective disorders' is applied to those disorders in which the main feature is a change of emotion: this change may be a raising or lowering of mood. Low mood is sometimes referred to as depression and it should really be reserved to describe a lowering of the mood which is serious enough to interfere with the normal functioning of the individual. We all feel low from time to time but hope that it will pass fairly quickly so that we are able to carry on with our lives. When the mood is high we call it hypomania or mania, the former being just slightly below the level of full-blown mania. Again, we all have peaks when we feel on top of the world but not to the extent that we act irrationally or misguidedly, nor do we usually break the rules of our society because we are uninhibited.

The affected disorders are classified as follows:

Psychoses	*Neuroses*
Manic-depressive psychosis (a) Depressive type (sometimes called endogenous depression) (b) Manic type (including hypomania) (c) Cyclical type (when the sufferer swings from depression to mania and back again, spending varying periods of time somewhere between the two extremes)	Reactive depression (sometimes called exogenous depression)

WHAT CAUSES DEPRESSION AND MANIA?

In Chapter 2 we identified numerous causes of mental ill-health. Genetic, neurochemical, cognitive (the way one thinks), personality and environmental causes have been identified. Sometimes the reason appears to be obvious, e.g. failing an examination, and this would be classed as a reactive depression since it is a reaction to something that has happened. But why does not everyone who fails an examination become depressed? You might say that it is because the examination is more important to one person than to another, but it could be that certain things actually predispose one person to respond to stress in a depressive way whilst another person is somehow protected from this response, perhaps through a different upbringing, way of thinking or personality. If we cannot identify an external cause for the depressed state it is referred to as endogenous, which means arising from within oneself. It is also classed as endogenous (a psychosis) if there are 'psychotic' features, i.e. being out of touch with reality, having hallucinations or delusions. But whatever the depression is called the fact remains that the individual is low in mood. There is no neurotic or reactive equivalent for mania. As has been mentioned, some individuals fluctuate between depression and mania, the manic-depressive disorder.

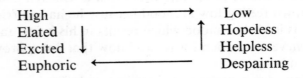

You will remember that in Chapter 1 a list of twenty positive health statements was introduced which you were asked to test on yourself; this approach is used again in the present chapter to illustrate the difficulties experienced by two patients, one whose mood is low and the other high.

Personal details   *Name:* Lorna Rossi
Age: 52
Religion: None
Civil status: Married
Reason for admission: Overdosed on prescribed antidepressants
Diagnosis: Depression

Name: James Foskett
Age: 52
Religion: None
Civil status: Married
Reason for admission: Physically violent toward GP who visited James at his wife's request. Abusive to neighbours and police. Threatening to kill his wife for betraying him.
Diagnosis: Hypomania

Lorna's problems	*James's problems*
I take a well-balanced diet and sufficient fluids to maintain normal weight and fluid/electrolyte balance	
Finds she has no appetite and cannot be bothered to eat food she has managed to cook for her family recently; has lost 2.5 kg in 6 months	Does not need food, according to him; has no time to waste anyway; tends to grab food and consume it very quickly, regardless of temperature; spills food and handles it inappropriately
I obtain sufficient rest and sleep to meet my body's physiological requirements and to feel refreshed	
Has not been sleeping well for weeks; finds she wakes up at 4 a.m. and cannot go back to sleep; feels permanently tired	Has only slept for a couple of hours each night for a week, but naps on and off during remainder of night; will not remain in bed when awake; likes others to be awake too
I take enough exercise to prevent the complications of inactivity	
Feels like doing nothing at all; housework, shopping, etc. all too much for her; tends to sit around all day even though there are things to do; feels like she is slowing down	On the move from early morning to night; does not like to sit down for any length of time; has been 'jogging' around the ward
I breathe adequately to meet my body's respiratory requirements	
No problems	Smoking as many cigarettes as he can get; usually only smokes ten a day; coughing quite a lot
I eliminate waste from my body comfortably	
Has not had her bowels open for three days, which is unusual for her and is concerning her	Has not has his bowels open for two days; laughing about being 'blocked up'
I achieve a state of pain-free physiological homeostasis	
Slightly nauseated and in a little discomfort due to her bowel problem	—
I appreciate my personal strengths and weaknesses realistically whilst maintaining an overall positive self-image	
Describes herself as 'a bit of a let-down'; feels she should be doing more but is letting it all mount up; complains of feeling really low at times and has a cry two or three times a day; often just feels nothing at all	Maintains 'I am the greatest'; says he is going to run ICI since he is a financial wizard; says he will invest money for the patients so they can 'make a killing on the market'
I achieve success and satisfaction in personal relationships, work and social activities	
Says everything is going wrong; thinks her marriage is only hanging together because of duty; no social outlets, although she used to belong to a church group	Embarrassing other patients and his family; sent off sick from work following an argument with his manager

continued on next page

continued

Lorna's problems	*James's problems*
I divide my time in such a way as to carry out all that is needed without undue pressure	
Lets housework get on top of her; just cannot summon up the energy to get anything done	Doing many things but finishing none; concentration minimal; highly distractable
I make realistic interpretations based on observations and information that I receive	
Minimizes positive aspects and maximizes negative aspects of her life; seems to generalize a lot and to make negative predictions based on little or irrational evidence	Thinks that everyone admires him because of his 'abilities'; believes he has been brought here to sort out the NHS before going on to ICI
I minimize danger to myself and others	
Has spoken to her husband about suicide; admits to thinking it would be a good way out	Does not bother where he puts his cigarettes; provokes other patients, endangering himself
I obtain pleasure in expressing thoughts and feelings in a manner which does not cause offence to others	
Finds it very difficult to get her thoughts together and to explain how she feels; believes nobody is interested and nobody could understand her feelings; long silences during conversations	Tactless and rude to others, including staff and his family; talks uninhibitedly about sex and masturbation, advocating sex between various patients on the ward as being 'therapeutic for them'; thoughts/speech in rapid succession; ideas seem only slightly related to each other
I find satisfaction through recreational/relaxational activities	
Has no recreational activities now and no energy to bother	Has recently indulged in much strenuous physical exercise; has started four new hobbies during the past month
I maintain an adequate and acceptable roof over my head	
Worries about money problems and the deteriorating state of her home, although these concerns are apparently unjustified	Has started to redecorate three rooms at once; according to him, is planning to convert his home into a show house for the public
I look forward to my future and am motivated to continue living	
Says life drags on and she cannot see things improving	Says life is wonderful for people like him
I set realistic goals and make appropriate decisions independently	
Cannot make even simple decisions for fear of them being wrong; dithers over everyday decisions, and gets into 'a state'	Decisions are questionable and show lack of judgement and an inability to appreciate the likely consequences

continued on next page

THE UPS AND DOWNS OF FEELINGS

continued

Lorna's problems	James's problems

I look after myself without having a rely on others	
Cares for own hygiene but has paid little attention to her appearance, saying she cannot be bothered anymore	Unkempt appearance; wearing odd combinations and colour coordinations

I satisfy my sexual needs within my cultural boundaries	
No interest in sex and has not had intercourse for five months	Uninhibited sexually; masturbating openly in the dormitory

I practise my own philosophy of life or religion	
Has always believed in 'putting on a good face' but cannot now	Freedom with touch and comments offend others; wife cannot see this as an illness but believes he is trying to hurt her

I function in the company of others in such a way as to satisfy myself and not unduly interfere with their functioning	
Socially isolated and friendless except for immediate family; finds it very hard to join in with others; usually rather shy	Causing considerable irritation and embarrassment to others; inappropriate behaviour resulting in aggressive responses from some

Helping Lorna

The aim, using this model, is to enable Lorna to convert her current statements into the positive statements in the list (our goal). Nursing staff will assist her where necessary, encouraging her to do as much for herself as possible. What she cannot do for herself they will do for her.

Problem 1
Provide small, frequent meals. Offer fluid substitutes, particularly nourishing drinks. Ensure the mealtime environment and atmosphere are conducive. Check weight fortnightly.

Problem 2
Hypnosedatives offered initially. Encourage warm bath prior to retiring and a warm drink taken to bed. Encourage her to go for a walk in the fresh air each day. Teach relaxation techniques and encourage their use in bed.

Problems 3, 9 and 16
Help Lorna structure her day by identifying what has to be done, e.g. having a wash, what needs to be done, e.g. bedmaking and what she would like to do, e.g. have her hair washed and trimmed. Help her to set realistic time-limits for these activities and identify strategies for achieving them. Encourage her to tick them off as they are done. Ensure time is built in for sitting thinking, 30 minutes for a nap on her bed, and some time with nothing special to do.

Problems 5 and 6

Will probably resolve themselves once Problem 1 is dealt with and she takes more exercise. If necessary, give two suppositories by 5th day. Explain most likely reason for her constipation to allay any illness worries she may have.

Problems 7, 8, 10, 14 and 19

Praise minor effort. Encourage Lorna to help in small ways. Point out her tendency to abstract selectively the negative aspects of herself and her day. Identify when she maximizes unimportant happenings. Ask her to keep a record of how she feels during the day and what situations and thoughts were occurring at the times of low mood. Arrange for her husband to help to validate their relationship and to reassure her.

Problems 11 and 15

Observe Lorna unobtrusively at this stage although one-to-one close observation may be necessary later. Assess degree of risk through monitoring her actions and conversation. Remember that people who talk about suicide carry out the act in around 60–70% of instances. Observe more closely during evenings and weekends and once some degree of improvement seems apparent. Take care with all potentially dangerous objects. To commit suicide one needs the will, the means and the energy—bear all of these in mind.

Problems 12 and 20

Allocate 30 minutes in the morning and again in the afternoon to be alone with Lorna. If no conversation is forthcoming, ask her to focus on one particular aspect of her life. Remember to try to introduce a positive aspect. Shared silences may be useful, as may touch, to communicate that you value her even though she is silent. Encourage her to participate in any group work going on in the ward. Emphasize that she does not have to join in verbally but that being there may help since others have had similar problems and felt the same. Try group work based on each member participating in discussion on a newspaper article. Help her express herself through art.

Problem 17

Reinforce all effort. Discourage her from remaining in night attire.

Problem 18

Make time available for husband. Assess his feelings. Offer help with any particular aspects of their relationship he may wish to discuss. May be appropriate later to suggest sex therapy if still necessary.

EXERCISE 1

> Once the initial life-preserving measures had been taken in the medical ward to which Lorna was initially admitted, which of the interventions identified under 'Helping Lorna' could have been implemented in this ward if the decision to transfer her to the psychiatric department had not been made? If there were any interventions you felt could not be realistically introduced in the medical ward what constraints would have applied?

EXERCISE 2

P. Vaughan, in *Suicide Prevention*, identified a group of people who harm themselves deliberately, were psychologically unstable and had disorganized lifestyles. They often repeated the act of harming themselves. He identified a second group who were stable and organized but who invested too much in one person or situation and were thus made vulnerable if that special person went away or the situation changed. Try to identify one person you have nursed in each of these categories. Think about what was done for them prior to their return to the community and then compare it with what you now feel, in retrospect, could and should have been done for them. Look especially at what was done to help them to deal with life events similar to those that precipitated the act, should these recur.

Helping James

EXERCISE 3

Below you will find a number of interventions, some of which would be appropriate when nursing James and some which would not. In the column on the right tick those which you feel would be useful nursing interventions.

Appropriate
Interventions

 1 Provide food which can be eaten 'on the move'.
 2 Give drinks which are very hot and sweet.
 3 Place him at a table with depressed patients for meals so that
   he will encourage them to eat.
 4 Sleep him in a dormitory rather than a single room.
 5 Encourage physical, energetic activities.
 6 Do not allow him to smoke.
 7 Agree with him that 'he is the greatest' to avoid an argument.
 8 Distract him from inappropriate behaviour by offering alternative
   activities.
 9 Assess when his concentration is lapsing and provide alternative
   activity.
10 Pretend you can follow his train of thought even when you cannot.
11 Allow him to masturbate when necessary, explaining to other
   patients that this is a natural act.
12 Give daily suppositories.

When you have completed this exercise, identify your reasons for choosing the actions you think are appropriate, and for rejecting the others. Check your responses against those given on p. 90.

REFERENCE

Vaughan, P. (1985) *Suicide Prevention*. PEPAR Publications.

FURTHER READING

Bowlby, J (1979) *Affectional Bonds*. London: Tavistock Publications.

Brooking, J. (ed.) (1986) *Psychiatric Nursing Research*. Chichester; John Wiley & Sons (see chapter on *Group Therapy with Women*, by Verona Gordon).

Brooking, J. & Minghell, E. (1987) Parasuicide. *Nursing Times*, 27 May.

Goodwin, J. (1986) Managing pregnancy-related depression. *Patient Care*, 39 March, 107–114.

Hauck, P. (1973) *Depression*. London: Sheldon Press.

Morgan, H. (1979) *Death Wishes? The Understanding and Management of Deliberate Self-harm*. Chichester: John Wiley & Sons.

Rippere, V. & Williams, K. (1986) *Wounded Healers*. Chichester: John Wiley & Sons (see *Wading Through the Mud*, written by a clinical psychologist).

Weissman, M. & Paykel, E. (1974) *The Depressed Woman*. Chicago: Phoenix Books — University of Chicago Press.

Chapter 6

Memory, Reality and Perception Problems

This chapter will cover two conditions that are classed as psychoses and in which problems of memory, reality and perception may be evident. You may remember that the psychotic disorders are divided into functional psychoses and organic psychoses. We shall look at organic psychoses in the form of acute brain syndrome (known also as delirium or confusional state) and chronic brain syndrome (dementia). Acute brain syndrome is a temporary, reversible, non-progressive condition and is seen, for example, following head injury, after an anaesthetic, as a consequence of therapy with certain drugs (particularly in the elderly), accompanying a high temperature, constipation or an infection. Chronic brain syndrome has an insidious onset, is progressive, irreversible and permanent.

In Chapter 2 we studied some of the causes of mental health problems. For the organic psychoses (psychoses in which there is demonstrable cerebral pathology) these include genetic factors, neurotransmitter deficiency, auto-immunity, impaired blood supply and poisons. Whatever the cause, the result is a loss of brain cells and as brain cells (neurons) do not multiply or regenerate the brain becomes smaller, its characteristic shape changes and the ventricles become enlarged. The individual has to function on less brain tissue.

Dementia can affect some people before they reach the age of 65 years and is then called presenile dementia. There are four types of presenile dementia as illustrated by the following case histories.

ALZHEIMER'S DISEASE

William Brown was 55 when his wife first noticed little changes in what he could do: small problems presented more difficulty than usual and his memory began to fail. He became very inflexible, and if pressured would become very angry. He did not accept that anything different was happening. Within five years William became a completely different person. He was quite unable to dress himself, was very excitable and had tremendous difficulty putting a sentence together or even finding a particular word. He was noticeably clumsy and unsteady on his feet, he failed to recognize members of his family and spent his days with a perplexed, agitated expression on his face as he wandered around, touching everything he found.

Key Features

Problem-solving difficulties
Memory impairment
Inflexibility of thought processes
Catastrophic reaction (anger when pressured)
Lack of insight
Inability to dress
Dysphasia
Agnosia
Apraxia
Disturbed gait
Hyperexcitability

PICK'S DISEASE

Lucy was in her early fifties when it was first remarked by her friends and family that she seemed to be showing a remarkable lack of interest in things that previously would have concerned her. She seemed to lack the initiative to do anything unless told to and did not really care whether she did it or not. She became incontinent at times and although she would have been horrified by this previously she made no fuss. She deteriorated over the next couple of years and her memory failed her more and more. She had no idea where she was and would wake up at night thinking it was daytime. Her family found that she would repeat words said to her quite happily but not initiate and sustain any real conversation, although she would ramble incomprehensibly. There was also a marked lack of muscle tone.

Key Features

Lack of concern or care
No initiative
Incontinent
Memory impairment
Variation in day/night pattern
Echolalia
Incomprehensible speech
Hypotonia

JACOB–CREUTZFELD'S DISEASE

Gordon had been employed as a draughtsman until he became ill when he was 56 years old. Within months of the first symptoms being noticed he was severely demented, being confused, disoriented, incontinent, unable to sustain any conversation and apparently unable to grasp the meaning of anything. He was a totally different person, being more irritable and irresponsible in the early days and, later on, totally degraded in his personal habits and hygiene. There was an early marked deficit in his ability to coordinate which had made him totally unable to do his job. His muscles, particularly in his legs, were atrophied and he made sudden involuntary movements. He also appeared not to see clearly and this, coupled with his difficult unsteady gait, led to numerous falls.

Key Features

Confused
Disoriented
Incontinent
Unable to grasp meanings
Personality change
Visual/spatial coordination poor
Myoclonia fasciculations and muscle-wasting
Unsteady gait
Failing eyesight

HUNTINGTON'S CHOREA

Mr J. was adopted when he was ten years old by the Rev. Wilson and his wife. He knew nothing of his parents since he had spent the previous seven years in an orphanage. Mr J. had an uneventful childhood and adolescence and married when he was 23. He and his wife both worked and were buying their home. They had one son. In 1979, when Mr J. was 35, Mrs J. began to find aspects of her husband's behaviour very trying. He would accuse her of being unfaithful to him and would watch her constantly. He was irritable and unpredictable and began to neglect himself, not shaving as often as he used to and not washing as frequently. He apparently began to forget where he had put things and would accuse his wife of taking them. He hit her on a number of occasions. Soon he developed odd little jerky movements in his limbs and he seemed unable to sit still while watching television. He frequently choked over his meals and people started to comment on the change in his gait. A doctor was consulted and a neurologist diagnosed the disorder. Within three years he was unable to walk except by lurching, feet wide apart, arms abducted and rolling side to side. These movements, coupled with sudden jerking of his arms and slow writhing movements of his head, neck and trunk, did not cease until he fell asleep. Within six years he was grossly demented, only mumbling incoherently, incontinent and confined to a specially adapted chair since his movements prevented him from staying in any other chair.

Key Features

Personality change
Suspicious
Jealous
Memory failure
Choreo-athetoid movements
Characteristic lurching gait
Speech difficulties
Choking

Senile dementia, which occurs after 65 years of age, is usually a multi-infarct dementia or an Alzheimer-type dementia.

SENILE DEMENTIA

Charles was 74 when his wife died and he went to live with his married daughter and her family. She knew he had problems which her mother had coped with but she did not realize the extent of them. He was quite dangerous, leaving the front door open and the gas on but unlit. He seemed to lack any insight into why people were concerned and would become very easily moved to tears but suddenly quite happy again. He could not always understand what was said to him and even though it was explained three or four times he did not seem to remember. He would wander around saying he was going to school, if asked, and would continually ask for the newspapers. His social behaviour coarsened and he would stuff food into his mouth with both hands and come out of the toilet without pulling up his trousers. He would hold long conversations with himself and ramble on incomprehensibly to others. He could become very resistive when it came to bedtime and his son-in-law lost his temper several times because, having undressed him and put him to bed, he would be found wandering around half-dressed and going to catch the school bus. He often called his son-in-law 'dad'.

EXERCISE 1

> Pick out ten key features from the example above. Imagine you are the married daughter who is looking after Charles. In what ways would each of the features you have identified affect your life and that of your family?

EXERCISE 2

Get together with a group of colleagues: each of you take one of the following roles and hold a family discussion about which of you is the best person to look after your aged demented parent (imagine that he is exactly like Charles in the case study). Try to identify the implications for whoever is chosen to care for the demented parent.

1 You are 35 years old, married with two children under ten years of age. Your husband is a solicitor and you look after the house and family. You live in the country and your husband commutes 10 miles each day to the nearest large town. You plan to return to teaching once your children get into secondary education.
2 You are single, 31 years old and lived with your parents until four years ago, when you moved to a flat in the city. It is in a very nice block with a porter and is ideally suited to your place of work. You are a fashion designer and doing very well. From time to time you have men friends to live with you although you are currently 'between boyfriends'.
3 You are 45 years old and recently divorced after 25 years of marriage. Your children are now away from home. You are an only son. You work as a school teacher and rent your flat from the council. You are at present undergoing a course of antidepressant drugs prescribed by your GP.
4 You are married to a man 20 years older than yourself (you are 40). He suffers from Parkinson's disease but is still active. You care for him at home and he has retired during the last year on health grounds. You have a small cottage in a village and your husband has had to give up driving which has isolated both of you since you do not drive. Your cottage has one bedroom upstairs and a huge lounge downstairs which used to be two rooms. The toilet is downstairs.

PLANNING CARE FOR CONFUSED PATIENTS

Reality Orientation and Reminiscence Therapy

Reality orientation (RO) is a rehabilitation technique which is used to help those who are confused, disoriented and experiencing memory impairment. Reminiscence therapy may be used separately but it is often included as part of a reality orientation programme. Twenty-four hour reality orientation involves every encounter being used to bring reality home; for example: 'Good morning Mr Jones, it's lovely this bright June morning. It's nearly 8.30 so if you'd like to get up, breakfast will be ready at 9 a.m.'. Or 'It's 12.30 Mr Jones, time for your lunch—are you coming into the dining room?' Both these examples orientate the individual to who he is, what time of day it is and what is about to happen.

Formal RO can take place in the classroom or other suitable setting and consists usually of a period of time spent concentrating on group work. The session begins with the participants introducing themselves; then a map may be used to identify the whereabouts of certain places, including the hospital ward, day centre or wherever the session is taking place. The environment should always limit confusion, where possible: for example, each room should be clearly marked with the occupant's name. Keeping personal possessions should be encouraged. Photographs and other mementos should be brought in and used to facilitate the recollection of past events because the past is part of present reality. Old pictures projected onto a screen can be discussed and old songs sung or played and talked about.

Safety

Many demented patients are prone to accidents because of their unsteady gait or carelessness, particularly if they smoke or have access to cooking facilities. It is important to remind them frequently of safety features and to remain vigilant at all times.

Communication

It is frightening and frustrating to be unable to understand or to be understood. Time and repetition are the keys to communicating with confused people: by standing in front of them, attracting their attention and keeping communication short and to the point, the message may be conveyed, although it will probably have to be repeated. There is no point in being annoyed when having to repeat a message because as far as the patient is concerned he is hearing it for the first time and will only feel bad because you seem unjustifiably to be irritated with him. It is important never to talk 'rubbish' to a patient and far better to point out to him that you cannot understand or follow what he is saying. It helps if you attempt to anticipate what it is he is trying to tell you and to put it into words for him, asking if that is what he means. It seems kind and easy just to go along with little statements such as 'I'm going to catch the train to work, now' but if this is not, in reality, what he is about to do then it should be pointed out gently that he no longer goes to work and that it would be better if he did something else, for example, coming with you to the kitchen to make tea. If the patient is resistive to attention it is often best to leave him alone for a while or to help him to do whatever he wishes and then explain to him why you wish to help him to do whatever it is *you* are trying to achieve with him, and try again. Sometimes another person may be able to accomplish what you cannot achieve. This is not usually a reflection of the relationship but merely that at that moment the patient is not responding to you or to your approach for some reason which it may or may not be possible to identify. Later, even that same day, you may be his best friend again and able to achieve all manner of things that others cannot.

SELF-EVALUATION—1

---

1 Name four types of presenile dementia.
2 Which of the above types is caused by a virus, and how is it transmitted?
3 How is Huntington's chorea transmitted and what chance would the children of someone with this disease have of suffering from it also?
4 Name four pathological cerebral changes that occur in dementia.
5 What is the difference between an organic and a functional psychosis?
6 What is meant by the following terms? apraxia
agnosia
confabulation
echolalia
choreo-athetoid movements

Answers will be found on p. 91.

A Problem with Reality

Reality is difficult to define. What is reality to me may not be reality to you. We can expect to share certain realities such as who we are, what we are wearing, who is in the room with us, and so on; however, once we begin to think about reality in terms of what is beautiful and what is ugly, what is nice and what is repulsive, we may then find that our realities differ. None of us is right and none is wrong, but we will probably not agree on the reality of the situation.

Martin's reality was certainly not shared by others. It is an example of a functional psychosis.

Name: Martin Frazer
Age: 27
Occupation: Unemployed (had several jobs after leaving university but has not worked for four years)
Diagnosis: Paranoid schizophrenia

Problems

1. Martin believed that he was being hunted by an alien force who had spies everywhere. The spies were in human guise and were capable of taking on the form of people familiar to him. This is termed a delusion, in that it is a false belief, not shared by others from the same cultural group and not amenable to rational explanation. Delusions may be of grandeur, poverty, guilt, or, as in this instance, persecution. Sometimes the individual believes that his bodily organs are changing in some way (somatic delusion) or even that he is dead (nihilistic delusion), even though he will carry on with his normal daily activities.

2. He heard the voices of these aliens when they were planning what they would do to him; this is called an auditory hallucination. A hallucination is a false sensory preception occurring in the absence of an objective stimulus and may affect any of the five senses, i.e. olfactory hallucination (smell), visual hallucination (sight), auditory hallucination (hearing), tactile hallucination (touch) and gustatory hallucination (taste).

3. When in conversation, Martin would stop suddenly in mid-sentence and go off at a tangent. He would use words which nobody could understand and claim that people were taking thoughts out of his head. It was very difficult to get a straight answer out of him since he would go round and round and off the point constantly. These symptoms indicate the thought disorder present in Martin: he stops in mid-sentence (thought blocking), makes up new words (neologisms), claims you take his thoughts (thought withdrawal) and misses going straight to the point (circumstantiality).

Nursing Approaches

In caring for Martin it was important that his false reality should not be reinforced and, therefore, nobody would say to him 'Good evening to you, Martin, and good evening to the aliens as well.' This would not be seen as a joke, nor would it be reality-based. Instead, when he was observed to be listening the nurse would distract him and try to involve him in some meaningful activity. The staff reinforced the point that although they appreciated how very worrying it must be to feel that the aliens were going to harm him, in fact nobody else believed this and there was no evidence at all that this was or ever could be the case. It was emphasized that this is the stuff of which science fiction films are made. All staff adopted the same approach so that he was not given conflicting views. When at times he became convinced that the staff were aliens, the same technique was used to deny this but it was important to make sure that he did not feel cornered or singled out in any way. It was essential to treat him in the same way as other patients. He was given as much freedom of choice as possible and allowed to select his food from the main trolley without any fuss. The staff tried to be as truthful as possible and when, for instance, he said he knew that they talked about him behind the office door they responded by saying that they discussed *every* patient since that was the purpose of the staff handover and that what was talked about was the progress and problems of each one.

Staff kept their conversations to the point and would refocus him when he went off the issue or when he seemed to be experiencing concentration difficulties. If he used a word that could not be understood this was pointed out to him and he would be asked either to try to use a word which they could all understand or to explain what he was referring to. He was told that staff were always there and that no harm would come to him. Although he was told he could come to them whenever he felt threatened by his voices or a situation on the ward, the staff tended to discourage him from spending a lot of time talking about the delusional content of his thoughts and would ask him to repeat what we had told him about these ideas or thoughts, for that was all they were.

SELF-EVALUATION—2

1 What is meant by a nihilistic delusion?
2 Define the term hallucination.
3 Name five types of hallucination.
4 What is meant by thought blocking?
5 What is meant by circumstantiality?

Answers will be found on p. 91.

FURTHER READING

Phillips, D. (1982) *Living with Huntington's Chorea*. London: Junction Books.
Stokes, G. (1986) *Wandering*: Winslow Press.
Stokes G. (1986) *Shouting and Screaming*: Winslow Press.
Trick, K. & Daisley, R. (1980) *Handbook of Psychogeriatric Care*. London: Pitman Medical.

Chapter 7

Alcohol and Drug-related Problems

EXERCISE 1

> Keep a diary of the amounts of the following substances that you use during a one-week period: coffee
> tea
> tobacco
> alcohol
> any other drug
> recording your behaviour under the following headings:
> 1 How much per day?
> 2 At what time or times of the day or night
> 3 The circumstances surrounding the activity, e.g. offered by another person, suddenly felt the urge, etc.

Add up your totals and, if possible, compare them with those of other people. Are you surprised at the amounts you have taken? Caffeine, for example, is a stimulant and each cup of tea or 'instant' coffee contains about 70 mg: fresh coffee contains double that amount. In a questionnaire produced by the North-West Thames Health Authority and reproduced in the training package *Working with Drug-users*, students were asked to decide from the following description of his symptoms what drug the individual is withdrawing from: 'The sufferer is tremulous and loses his self-command; he is subject to fits of agitation and depression; he loses colour and has a haggard appearance.' The answer is caffeine!

THEORETICAL ASPECTS

It is difficult to establish how many people in the UK misuse alcohol and other drugs. If we were to consider only the number of notified addicts, i.e. those people abusing controlled drugs who are notified to the Home Office under the Misuse of Drugs (Notification of and Supply to Addicts) Regulations 1973, we might be led to believe that there are only around 7000 addicts. Most drugs agencies believe that a realistic figure is more likely to be ten times that number. In *Drug Misuse* (1985), a pamphlet prepared by the Central Office of Information, the estimated figure for people using cannabis is given as one million. It is very hard to determine the number of youngsters who abuse solvents because many do so on a very temporary or occasional basis. However, we do know that nearly 100 children died from solvent abuse in 1983. To identify how many people abuse alcohol it is necessary first to establish whether we are looking at alcoholics, problem drinkers or heavy drinkers. The World Health Organization defines alcoholism as 'those excessive drinkers whose dependence on alcohol has attained such a degree that it causes a noticeable mental disturbance or an interference with their bodily or mental health, their inter-personal relations and their smooth social and economic functioning.' DHSS figures reveal that in England and Wales 9%, and in Scotland 20%, of admissions to mental hospitals are alcohol-related. This obviously represents the tip of an iceberg. Some alcohol abusers are easy to identify. For example, some people have an abstinence problem which simply means that in order to function reasonably well they need to keep 'topped up' with alcohol, and so long as they can get a drink when they need it they may appear to be coping. Others have a control problem and although they may go for periods without alcohol they will over-indulge once they restart: this group will appear drunk. Some groups are a combination of both.

Whichever figures we accept, it is obvious that there is a growing problem. All the substances we are discussing will cause physical and/or psychological dependence which is characterized by withdrawal symptoms or a craving when the substance is unavailable to the body and mind. Some would argue that solvents and LSD, for instance, produce neither but there is often a desire to repeat the behaviour and always the danger that the user may 'progress' to something 'addictive'. Tolerance develops with many substances and this means that more is needed as time goes by in order to achieve the same effect. Tolerance develops even with hallucinogenic mushrooms.

The table on pages 48 and 49 gives an idea of the substances and their effects.

In searching for the reasons why one individual uses these agents appropriately and another abuses them we have to look at the interplay of three factors, namely the individual himself, the environment he lives in, and the agent itself. Certain individuals seem more prone to alcohol abuse, and twin studies by people such as Goodwin in the 1970s revealed what seemed to be a genetic factor. It is important to look at children who have been adopted away from alcoholic parents because it would be difficult to know whether it was a genetic factor that influenced the development of the disease (if, in fact, it is a disease) or the effect of the environment they were brought up in. Some say that alcoholics metabolize alcohol differently from non-alcoholics and that as a consequence they are more prone to its addictive effects. People who abuse substances often show a particular type of personality that finds frustration very hard to take. Some lack confidence and are more prone to peer-group pressure, while others are shy and feel inferior, needing the boost and release of inhibitions that these substances may offer, at least temporarily. The environment plays a part, especially with regard to availability of the agent. If you live and work in a climate where drugs and alcohol are the norm then you are more likely to be able to obtain them easily. Barmen, for example, have a high rate of alcoholism, as do businessmen who entertain a lot. Alcohol is everywhere and glamorized to some extent by the media. Drugs may not be glamorized but their antisocial aspects may attract, coupled with the relief from the real world which they may offer.

Substance	Therapeutic use	Desired effect when misused	Usual mode of administration	Withdrawal symptoms	Treatment notes
Narcotics: Diamorphine (heroin) Morphine Pethidine Methadone (Physeptone) Dipipanone (Diconal)	Analgesics Anti-diarrhoea Cough-suppressant	Warm, content, happy, a dreamy detachment	Oral Injected Sniffed Smoked	Yawning, sweating, shaking, sneezing, runny nose and eyes, abdominal pain, anorexia, gooseflesh, nausea, vomiting, diarrhoea	Controlled Drugs Only specially licenced doctors may prescribe heroin or Diconal for addicts. Usual treatment is to replace heroin with methadone and reduce that. Some authorities encourage 'cold turkey' withdrawal
Hypnosedatives: a) Barbiturates such as: Amylobarbitone (Tuinal) Quinalbarbitone (Seconal) Amylobarbitone sodium (sodium amytal)	To induce sleep Anticonvulsants Control withdrawal symptoms	Relaxed carefree feelings	Oral Suppositories Injected	Delirium, psychotic state, convulsions, twitching, irritability, sleeplessness	Controlled drugs Gradual withdrawal under supervision
b) Non-barbiturates such as: Nitrazepam (Mogadon) Flurazepam (Dalmane) Chlormethiazole (Heminevrin)		Usually prescribed and unintentionally dependence develops			Prescription only
Minor tranquillizers: Diazepam (Valium) Chlordiazepoxide (Librium)	Relief of anxiety	Usually prescribed and unintentionally dependence develops	Oral	Anxiety, insomnia, nausea, vomiting, confusion, convulsions, tremor	Gradual withdrawal. Modified narcosis may be offered

Drug	Legitimate uses	Effects	Method of use	Dependence	Legal status and comments
Stimulants:					
a) Amphetamine type: Dexamphetamine (Dexedrine) Methylphenidate (Ritalin)	To relieve pathological sleepiness, Reduces appetite Relieves depression	Euphoria. Greater capacity to work. Freedom from worry. Feelings of well-being. May be mixed with heroin (speedball) and taken in 'runs' (frequent injection)	Oral Injected Sniffed	Psychological dependence Depression and tiredness on withdrawal	Controlled drugs Paranoid psychois lasting for months may occur
b) Cocaine	Local anaesthetic			Psychological dependence	Controlled drug Sniffing cocaine destroys nasal septum
Hallucinogenics: Lysergic acid diethylamide (LSD) Phencyclidine (PCP) Magic mushrooms (e.g. Liberty Cap)	Occasionally for research	Perceptual changes Enhanced awareness Euphoria	Oral	Desire to repeat the experience only With mushrooms tolerance develops very rapidly	Controlled drugs (even mushrooms once prepared for this type of use) Prone to accidents due to judgement errors. Psychotic behaviour possible
Cannabis (hashish or marihuana)		Calm, relaxed state. Hallucinations	Smoked		
Solvents: Glue, petrol, surgical spirit, felt pens	Legitimate uses are obvious	Euphoria. Lightheadedness. Feeling of power and superhuman ability. Hallucinations called 'dreams'	Sniffed	A desire to repeat the experience only	Usually a transient episode which rarely continues after 16 yrs A full programme of activities with control from respected adults is the usual approach

Sources

All drugs may be obtained by the following methods: legitimate prescription; sold on the 'black-market'; given by a 'friend'; stolen including obtained by deceit; bought over the counter.

Controlled drugs

Possession is not as serious in the eyes of the law as trafficking. For a drug in Class A of the Misuse of Drugs Act 1971 the penalty for possession is a maximum of 7 years and for trafficking 14 years; for possession of a Class C drug it is 2 years and 5 for trafficking. The Medicines Act 1968 specifies that certain drugs are to be supplied by prescription only.

EXERCISE 2

Test your knowledge of substance abuse by answering 'true' or 'false' to each of the following statements:

1 Alcohol consumption is measured in units: 1 unit of alcohol is equivalent to one glass of whisky or one pint of beer.
2 The legal limit for alcohol in the blood is 17 mmol/litre of blood (80 mg/100 ml).
3 Alcohol is metabolized in the liver.
4 Women usually need less alcohol than men to become intoxicated because they have less water in their bodies and are generally smaller.
5 Food in the stomach slows the rate of absorption of alcohol.
6 There are more male alcoholics than female.
7 Alcohol is a cerebral stimulant.
8 Mainlining refers to injecting a substance subcutaneously.
9 Alcoholism affects all social and racial groups equally.
10 The chief danger of solvent abuse is the method which is used to take it.

Answers are to be found on p. 91.

Case History: Chasing the Dragon

The Customs Officer's Account

Somewhere in Pakistan there is a farmer who grows opium poppies of his acre of land. He sells his crop to a man with a factory which can process it into heroin. It is a profitable crop for the farmer. The factory owner sells it to an importer for ten times the price he paid for it. The importer pays a courier to bring it into Britain in his suitcase, in a false compartment in his car or even in his stomach, to be retrieved later. The importer sells it to a distributor for double or sometimes treble what he paid and it ends up on the streets at nearly 100 times the price the farmer was paid. The maximum sentence for trafficking is 14 years but the money involved makes it worth the risk for many people. The British government pays millions of pounds in an attempt to persuade the farmer to substitute an alternative crop in Pakistan.

The Addict's Account

When I was 14 years old I started on the glue. Everyone at school was doing it and, anyway, I was curious. I didn't touch anything else until I was 16 when I was given my first turn-on [cannabis cigarette]. I used it pretty regularly from then on and gradually I started taking other bits and pieces like the odd Tuinal, or a Diconal, if I could get it. My dad threw me out just after my 17th birthday. He said he didn't want the police round anymore. I moved in with mates and they used to let me score some smack [get some heroin] off them when they had any to spare. By the time I was 20 I was using it regularly but I didn't like the needle. Some blokes really enjoyed sticking themselves but they got lumps in their arms and some of them had lost fingers. One guy had lost his leg. One of the girls used to mix it with vinegar which is supposed to make you really buzz but she had a great big abscess from doing it.

For me it's best when I chase the dragon [put the heroin powder on a piece of tin foil and heat it, inhaling the smoke through a plastic straw]. I've given up two or three times but then something starts me again, like maybe I have a row with someone who offers me something cheap. Someone got a script [prescription] for some barbs [barbiturates] last week and gave me a few. I've got nothing else to do really but I would like to come off. I couldn't do cold turkey [have nothing to prevent the withdrawal symptoms] 'cause I've seen guys really screwed up. This time I had a row with the girl whose flat we were living in and her boyfriend threw me out. I didn't have my stuff with me and he wouldn't let me back in so I was really strung out [suffering withdrawal symptoms] so I went to the casualty department and they sent for this bloke from some voluntary agency.

The Psychiatrist's Account

When I saw Robert at the treatment centre he was in a pretty bad way physically since he had been unable to get a fix for nearly 48 hours. He was accompanied by a worker from a local drug project who was able to offer accommodation temporarily. Robert was homeless and only had £1.25 on him. He expressed a desire to come off heroin but had failed to do so previously. He was asking for relief from the symptoms he was experiencing. I decided that it would be better to maintain him on methadone until a place could be found for him as an in-patient. I arranged for him to collect his daily dose from a local chemist and wrote out a prescription accordingly and sent it off. I took some blood to check what he was taking because he denied using a needle but there was evidence of fairly recent use. Obviously now we check for hepatitis B and the AIDS virus since, according to one study by Peutherer *et al.* (1985) about 90% of drug abusers who inject have the hepatitis virus and about 5% the HIV virus associated with AIDS.

The Charge Nurse's Account (Drug Dependence Treatment Unit)

As soon as Robert was admitted he was given a standard contact which included total abstinence from any drug unless prescribed in this unit. It also prohibited visitors for the first three weeks of his stay. During this three-week period we administered methadone (Physeptone) in syrup form. Gradually the amount of methadone is reduced and eventually completely withdrawn. Detoxification is only the start for any addict. We worked on his physical state and Robert was certainly a physical wreck. It was important to teach him how to relax and we placed a lot of emphasis on diversional and occupational therapy activities. As clients progress through the programme they go on outings with staff and then start to help with the work of the unit like cleaning or preparing the evening meal. Each morning Robert attended the group meeting to talk about any problems and to look at ways of dealing with life without drugs. He, like all the others, had an individual counsellor who, in his case, was a nurse. It could be anyone from the team. He had to focus on why he took drugs and what sort of problems he might have when he left the unit. We aim to send people out after twelve weeks, drug-free and with the ability to stay off drugs. There is a very high failure rate and more than half will abuse some substance or other back in the community. For Robert we decided to send him to a hostel run along therapeutic community lines and where they continue the work started in this unit. He was keen to go even though he knew it would be pretty strict there.

The Social Worker's Account

My main role was to assess his social situation. It was actually rather bleak and it was obvious to me that he would need a lot of willpower to return to the community he came from and stay off drugs. He had no fixed address and would probably return to the area he had come from where his friends were. They were all still abusing drugs. He was typical of so many young men of his age from a working-class background with little positive that he could see in his future. He had used drugs as a way of hitting back at the society which seemed to promise so much but give so little. He was actually part of something, for a change, when he was taking drugs rather than just on the outside looking in. This is what Cohen (1956) called 'status frustration'. With his permission I got in touch with his family but they really did not want any further contact with him. They were worried about the influence he might have on his younger brother. He has no criminal record yet but has stolen, mainly shoplifting, to support his habit. I don't think he has ever been in a position to supply drugs to others since he has a job scraping together what he needs for himself. Even some of the people he shared with in the last house said that he really wasn't fussy what he mixed and would take anything anyone offered him. They considered him to be easily led with a tremendous lack of self-confidence.

Case History: 'Another Little Drink Won't Hurt'

The Ward Sister's Story

We admitted Sarah from the accident and emergency department around 3 p.m. that afternoon. She had fallen down a flight of stairs in a local shopping centre and, by all accounts, had lost consciousness. We commenced neurological observations but really she was OK except that she was very tearful about the whole event. She gave us the telephone number of her son who lived about 20 miles away and although we got through to him he didn't seem very interested. In fact, he said, 'Well what do you expect', which I thought was a bit funny. I asked if he would visit his mother since we would be keeping her in at least overnight. He said that he might but doubted it. Sarah had a strange attitude towards the staff in that she was slightly hostile to any questioning. She refused any supper and said that she wanted to go home at 8 p.m. She was distinctly agitated and restless although we asked her to remain in bed. Her hands shook visibly as she removed the bits and pieces from her shopping bag and replaced them about four times. She had no temperature although she appeared flushed and was slightly sweaty. When I went off duty I asked the night nurse to keep an eye on her because I thought she was possibly concussed. When I came on duty the next morning the night staff had had a terrible night with her. About 3 a.m. she started calling out and resisting all attempts to get her back to bed. They said it was as if she were terrified and they had tried to reassure her about where she was but she didn't seem to take it in. The duty doctor had been called and had prescribed chlorpromazine which was given intramuscularly to calm her. The cot sides were put up and she was placed in the observation room before I came on. When she opened her eyes around 10 a.m. her first words were: 'Give me a drink will you, love,' Nurse asked her what she would like and was told, 'Gin, if you've got any'. She was very unhappy and amongst all the tears she told us she had tried to kill herself and that she had thrown herself under a bus the previous day. The senior house officer from the psychiatric department was asked to visit, which he did, but she refused his offer of admission. Then a community psychiatric nurse came over and had a long talk with her. Eventually she agreed and was transferred to the psychiatric unit that afternoon as an emergency.

Sarah's Treatment Programme

1 She was detoxified using chlormethiazole starting at 2 g per day and decreasing over ten days to 250 mg.
2 She was given a contract stipulating no drink in the unit and none to be taken when outside or on leave. The programme lasts for six weeks.
3 Sarah had a well-balanced diet with plenty of fluids and Parentrovite injections initially, followed by Orovite tablets.
4 Group therapy was commenced after the two-weeks detoxification period because during the first two weeks she was expected to remain on bed rest.
5 Participation in an occupational therapy programme was encouraged so that she should have plenty with which to occupy her mind.
6 In her particular case, controlled drinking was not offered as an alternative to abstinence since she showed signs of liver damage and it was generally agreed by everyone, including Sarah, that it would be too difficult for her at this stage.

7 We spent a lot of time trying to help her to come to terms with the situation she found herself in and with the future, and how to face it without a drink.

8 She was helped to explore her reasons for drinking, the pattern and routine of her drinking and thus anticipate danger times once she was discharged.

9 She was given Antabuse (disulfiram) and after two weeks we gave her a small amount of alcohol just to check that we had the dose right. (If a patient receives the correct amount of Antabuse she will experience such symptoms as sweating, nausea, headache and tachycardia, and appear flushed.)

10 It was important to establish whether Sarah was depressed because of her drinking or drinking because of her depression. Either way, all staff were made aware of her suicide potential.

11 She was introduced to Alcoholics Anonymous during the six weeks that she was with us, so that attending meetings had become a habit before her discharge.

12 We tried to re-establish links with her son and daughter but both were unwilling.

13 Before discharging any patients, we like to ensure that they have somewhere to go to, money coming in and something to occupy them. They are all followed up by a community nurse from this unit who specializes in alcohol abuse. When discharging Sarah we warned her of the dangers of drinking whilst taking Antabuse and informed her that the effect of a tablet taken on one day lasts for up to four days. She was told that if she had any difficulty she could contact her community nurse and she was given an out-patient appointment for two weeks' time.

EXERCISE 3

1 When Sarah was admitted to the medical ward what signs should have given staff the clue to her alcohol problem?

2 What is chlormethiazole and why is it given in decreasing doses over ten days only?

3 Which vitamins are to be found in Parentrovite?

4 What is meant by 'controlled drinking' and how is it achieved?

5 Sarah did not just wake up one day and find herself to be alcoholic. Try to describe in a few sentences how someone might progress from being a social drinker to become an alcoholic and how her behaviour might change along the way.

Answers will be found on p. 92.

REFERENCES

Cohen, A. (1956) *Delinquent Boys*. Harmondsworth: Penguin Books.
Feutherer, J. *et al.* (1985) HTLV III virus in Edinburgh drug addicts (now known as HIV virus). *Lancet*, **16**, 11.
Goodwin, D., Schulsinger, F., Hermanson, L., Guze, J. & Winokur, G. (1973) Alcohol problems in adoptees. *Archives of General Psychiatry*, **28**, 238–243.

FURTHER READING

DHSS & Welsh Office (1985) *Drug Misuse—A Basic Briefing*. London: HMSO.
Gay, M. (1986) Drug and solvent abuse in adolescents. *Nursing Times*, 29 January, 34–35.
Goodwin, D. (1981) *Alcoholism: The Facts*. Oxford University Press.
Merrill, E. *Sniffing Solvents*. PEPAR.

Chapter 8

Diet-related Disorders

EXERCISE 1

Take any women's magazine and count in it the number of women of about size 10/12 who are modelling any product; compare this number with that of similar women of 16/18.

FOOD

Food is a significant substance in our lives. We show our love by offering it and by taking great care to produce it and present it nicely. We create social situations around it. Food can be used as a weapon from an early age because by rejecting offered food we can worry or reject the person who offers it.

SHAPE AND SIZE

Dieting is a common activity in Western society. Many people, women in particular, will at some stage in their lives try to reduce their weight by reducing their food intake. In most cases this is either a short-lived activity with varying degrees of success, or a long-term behaviour pattern with occasional lapses such as at Christmas. Our society is particularly concerned with the shape of the female form and this is reflected in the examples of desirable womanhood which the media offer us, in the products of the fashion industry and in the aids which are manufactured to help us in our quest for slimness. Our body image, that mental picture we have of what we look like, affects our self-image and our self-image affects the way we relate to other people. If we feel bad about the way we look we lack confidence, and this is reflected in our relationships. Our body image is affected by what people say about the way we look and by the values and attitudes of others, particularly during our early years. Body image may be altered by all kinds of surgery, by medical conditions such as arthritis, by having to use aids such as spectacles or a walking stick and by the ageing process, as well as in anorexia nervosa. Women are encouraged to be 'feminine' with all its implications. Oakley (1980) identifies the recurrent theme of self-doubt regarding self-worth and the capacity to control what happens to oneself. Controlling food intake is one thing that a woman can control in her life.

Anorexia nervosa is an extreme form of dieting resulting, in extreme cases in self-starvation. The lowest body weight known to the author was a 19-year-old girl weighing 2st 6lb (15.4 kg) but she had suffered from the disorder since early adolescence and her growth was generally stunted. Bulimia nervosa is a chaotic form of eating characterized by overeating (bingeing) and self-induced vomiting to control consequent weight gain. The two conditions may exist separately or may occur one after the other in the same individual.

Anorexia Nervosa

This disorder has existed for generations, although it was not until the 1870s that Sir William Gull and Professor Lasègue coined the phrase. Most sufferers are under twenty years of age, female and intelligent. There are numerous theories as to the cause but most revolve around either the difficulties of growing up and taking on adult responsibilities, disturbed relationships within the family, particularly with the mother, or something to do with the adolescent struggle for independence. To grow up means that one has to become an adult and can no longer escape the restrictions which that role entails. Many sufferers are profoundly depressed and may even be suicidal. Morgan & Russell estimate that 5% of sufferers will die from anorexia nervosa and its complications. For some of the remaining 95% the disorder will become chronic.

Bulimia Nervosa

Bulimia nervosa has also been recognized for a very long time. At Roman orgies huge quantities of food were consumed and vomited. However, it was not until the 1970s that Professor Christopher Fairbairn began to realize the extent of the problem and put an advertisement in a women's magazine asking women to tell him if they had ever controlled their weight by self-induced vomiting. Nine hundred women replied and of these, 700 returned the questionnaire he sent them. The bulimia sufferer is typically a female over twenty years old who controls her weight in this manner whilst still being able to function socially, including eating out with friends, and often her problem goes completely unnoticed. She is likely to buy and consume huge quantities of food, particularly of foods forbidden in diets, i.e. carbohydrates. She may incur large debts in order to buy all this food. She then induces vomiting by putting her fingers down her throat but later can induce vomiting simply by controlling her breathing and throat and stomach muscles. By bringing back the food she undoes the terrible thing she has done and this allays some of the guilt and disgust which she feels having 'made a pig of herself'. The behaviour may be repeated occasionally, at spaced intervals or on a regular daily basis. Purgatives may be used excessively to get rid of any food that has managed to escape the vomiting. Problems result from the alteration in electrolyte balance which vomiting brings about, from the acidity of the stomach contents eroding dental enamel and from the financial consequences of their behaviour. Treatment is usually through the introduction of control into the sufferer's life and thus preventing the behaviour whilst diverting her thinking through relaxation training and occupational therapy. Although it is difficult to establish why the behaviour occurs, counselling and social skills training, including assertiveness training, may help.

Case History: 'It's just a phase she's going through—it will pass'

Louise was, according to her father, 'a lovely podgy baby'. She had big dimples and chubby little legs which, apparently, 'would have done credit to a centre-half'. According to her mother she was always such a good child, trying hard at school, neat, tidy and interested in her appearance, which was not so for all her school friends. This pleased her mother and she was happy that she had no trouble from Louise. When she was 14 she, like many of her classmates, started dieting and instead of wanting cakes and biscuits she asked for salads. This was seen by her mother as a step in the right direction. Her mother had fought for years against the onslaught of middle-aged spread. Louise dieted on and off during the years leading up to the GCE examination, which she passed with 7 'O' levels. In the sixth form she worked harder and gradually her social life became more and more restricted and her friends no longer came to visit. This pleased her mother, who praised her daughter for studying: however, her mother complained constantly about her poor eating, and meal times became a battleground. These would end regularly with her mother shouting at her to show a bit more appreciation for what she did, like cooking and cleaning all day, and her father telling her to get up and out of his sight if all she could do was play around with good food, or with Louise bursting into tears and running up to her room. Her mother was really pleased one day when she found Louise eating a packet of chocolate biscuits, and when she heard her vomiting soon afterwards assumed that Louise, not having eaten properly for a long time, had eaten the biscuits too quickly. But the biscuit episode did not mark the end of the dieting since battle recommenced at the next meal. Her father commented once that he thought she was a bit skinny but she replied that she was fat really. Although her mother, who had not seen her daughter naked since the age of about 11 years, had failed to notice her weight-loss she did notice that Louise had stopped having periods. Although Louise denied that she was pregnant she was taken to the family doctor who, after spending 20 minutes alone with her, called in her mother and said that Louise would have to see a specialist who, much to her mother's horror, turned out to be a psychiatrist. Louise weighed 6st 4lb (39.9 kg), which shocked her mother because the big baggy jumpers she habitually wore had hidden this fact.

State on Admission

Every bone in Louise's body stood out, and her back was covered with the down-like hair known as lanugo hair. Her temperature, pulse and blood pressure were all lower than normal and her hands and feet were cold to the touch and slightly cyanosed. Although she had a pretty face her hair was dull and dry with noticeable split-ends, and she looked rather haggard.

Planning Care for Louise

Louise's problems were identified as follows:

1 Refusal to eat a normal, balanced diet.
2 Reluctance to talk about her feelings regarding her current situation or family relationships, although obviously distressed when the topic is raised.
3 Unsteady on her feet and dizzy at times, although she says she feels fine.
4 Very anxious about her future life including job prospects and role expectations.

Two other problems were identified once Louise had been in hospital for a while, namely:

5 Difficulty in communicating her needs and wishes in a straightforward manner.
6 Sees herself as useless, ugly and fat.

It was also apparent that her parents had a particular problem in accepting that Louise was ill since they felt it was a way of getting back at them (they could not say what she was getting back at them for) and they were very concerned about the stigma of their daughter being a patient in a psychiatric hospital.

EXERCISE 2

Try to think of nursing interventions which might help to resolve Louise's problems identified above and compare your answers with what was actually done in the psychiatric unit.

Problems 1 and 3

Louise was placed on bed rest in a side room and a programme of rewards in exchange for food eaten and consequent weight gain was commenced. The rewards were given from a list of things that she would like to have or do such as being able to watch her favourite television programme or have her knitting brought in. A target weight was set, using a standard height and weight chart, at which she would be discharged home. A commode was placed in the room and this prevented her from going to the toilet to dispose of food, which was a possibility. She was expected to eat all the food given to her since it had been carefully measured and items she did not normally enjoy eating had been excluded as far as possible. Louise was weighed weekly wearing only a nightdress. All staff were made aware of the possibility that she might attempt to hide food or falsify her weight in some way. She was given a copy of her own weight chart and the list of agreed rewards and the weight at which she would get each reward.

Problems 2, 4 and 6

Every day one of the nurses in the team caring for her would set aside an hour to sit with Louise and let her talk about whatever she wished. The nurses encouraged her to talk about relationships, the current situation and her future. Every opportunity was taken to reinforce the reality of her size and to help her to see herself in a more positive light. When she talked about being fat, usually accompanied by floods of tears, staff would tell her that her weight was well below normal, as had been established when she was first admitted, and then try to get her to focus on the effect dieting had had on her life or what 'size' really meant to her. She was encouraged to anticipate the future positively and without anorexia nervosa.

Problem 5

Louise was discouraged from asking indirectly for things or from trying to get staff to comply with her wishes even though these were not in line with the generally agreed approach. Whenever they felt that she was using an indirect method of communication, or that she was trying to manipulate a situation or be dishonest, staff would point this out. They would endeavour to help her to verbalize what she was really trying to say.

Apart from their usual visits, her parents were interviewed on three occasions; during these sessions the treatment regime was explained and their cooperation sought. It was important to help them to resolve their feelings about Louise, her problems and her hospitalization. Family therapy was to begin following discharge and Louise was introduced to Anorexic Aid, a self-help group, in the hope that she would continue to attend after discharge.

Evaluation of Nursing Interventions

After numerous ups and downs, good days and bad days, battles and reconciliations, Louise gained her target weight and was discharged home. The community nurse says that Louise has got a job as a nanny in Scotland and will be leaving home later in the year. Louise's parents had agreed to her leaving school and seemed to accept that this might be a good move and that she could always study for the two 'A' levels she was taking at some other time. Louise had managed to eat a somewhat controlled normal diet since discharge and had maintained her weight at 8st 8lb (54.43 kg).

SELF-EVALUATION

1 What is the likely mortality rate for sufferers of anorexia nervosa?
2 What behaviour typifies bulimia nervosa?
3 Describe six clinical features which might suggest anorexia nervosa.
4 Try to put yourself in Louise's place. Write an account of how you think she feels about her mother and father from the information you have been given about the family and her upbringing.
5 Could Louise have been treated in a medical ward? What difficulties might have been encountered if this had been the case? Could the interventions carried out in the psychiatric unit have been carried out in a medial ward. Discuss this with your colleagues.

Answers to Questions 1 and 2 will be found on p. 92. The answer to Question 3 can be found by referring to the main text of the chapter.

REFERENCES

Oakley, A. (1980) *Women Confined: Towards a Sociology of Childbirth*. London: Martin Robertson.
Fairbairn, C. & Cooper, P. (1984) The clinical features of bulimia nervosa. *British Journal of Psychiatry*, **144**, 238.
Russell, G. (1979) Bulimia nervosa. An ominous variant of anorexia nervosa. *Psychological Medicine*, **9**, 429.

FURTHER READING

Bond, M. (1982) Self-awareness. *Nursing Mirror*, **155** (13) 26.
Bruch, H. (1973) *Eating Disorders*. London: Routledge & Kegan Paul.
Dally, P. & Gomez, J. (1980) *Obesity and Anorexia Nervosa. A Question of Shape*. London: Faber & Faber.
Logue, A. (1986) *The Psychology of Eating and Drinking*: Freeman.
Salter, M. (1983) Towards a healthy body image. *Nursing Mirror*, **157** (11) (Supplement).

Chapter 9

Aggression

EXERCISE 1

Watch television for four hours during one evening. Count the number of times that aggressive behaviour is portrayed. In each example decide whether the aggressive act was purely to hurt or destroy or whether it served another purpose, e.g. to obtain something or to please someone. Identify what precipitated it and make a note of the body posture, facial expression and any other type of non-verbal behaviour that accompanied it. If possible, get a colleague to watch the same programme independently and compare notes the next day.

THEORETICAL ASPECTS

Aggression is sometimes defined as behaviour that is intended to damage. The term 'violence' is sometimes used instead. It may be purely to inflict suffering (hostile aggression) or may be to achieve another purpose (instrumental aggression): robbery with violence is an example of the latter type. It may be directed towards objects or people or animals and may be verbal or physical; it usually accompanies frustration, irritation, crossness, anger or rage. Generally speaking, the stronger the emotional arousal the more likely the aggressive behaviour but many factors determine whether aggression is the way we manifest an emotion. Most human beings seem to have the ability to control the expression of aggressive behaviour to some extent. We consider such things as the situation we find ourselves in, who or what the object of our aggression is, what the consequences might be and what was effective the last time we found ourselves in a similar situation.

Psychologists and others have studied aggression for many years but, as yet, there is little agreement about their findings. Some people believe that aggression is an instinct possessed by all animals, including humans, and all that is needed to release this behaviour is a trigger. Others, following Sigmund Freud's ideas, believe that everyone must express aggression since within all of us there are instinctive driving forces towards both pleasure and destruction. When our drive towards pleasure is thwarted, frustration occurs. If we cannot destroy ourselves we must damage or destroy others.

60

It has been shown that stimulation of the particular part of the brain called the hypothalamus can result in violence. Some individuals with brain damage show an increased tendency towards violence. At one time it was believed that men who had an extra Y chromosome in their genetic make-up showed an increased tendency to be aggressive, but this was later proved to be false by Owen (1973). The male hormone testosterone has been linked with aggressiveness.

Then we have the people who prefer to pay more attention to the social aspects of aggression, following the work of Bandura. It has been shown that we imitate behaviour witnessed in 'models', either real-life examples, such as a parent, or mass media examples such as violent television programmes. This imitation is particularly strong if the aggressive act results in reward rather than punishment, e.g. you get away with it or you are praised for it. Paterson *et al.* (1967) showed how true this is in childhood aggression. Aggression is sometimes socially acceptable and highly regarded, e.g. war heroes or vigilantes such as that portrayed by Charles Bronson in the films *Death Wish I* and *II* when he, single-handedly, kills numerous street muggers in retaliation for the murder of his wife years before. In the film he is hailed as a hero of the people and even the police have a sly respect for him. When aggression is used to protect the weak it is called 'prosocial agression'.

Some theorists believe that aggression is simply a drive that must be satisfied when we encounter frustration because our behaviour is directed towards a goal and if we are prevented from achieving that goal we experience frustration (Dollard *et al.* 1935). There are those who believe that this aggressive drive can be satisfied through watching others being aggressive. They feel that by watching aggression you actually satisfy your need for it but without having to be aggressive yourself: this is referred to as vicarious satisfaction. But there are an equal number of people who would say that this does not reduce one's own drive but in fact increases the likelihood of violence (Steuer *et al.* 1971). It was demonstrated by Eron *et al.* (1972) that little boys who watched a lot of violent television by choice developed into aggressive adults. Some people believe that because we all have angry feelings these should be released through aggression and that this will therefore relieve our angry feelings in the same way that when we are hungry eating food relieves our hunger. However, Green & Quanty (1977) showed that this was untrue and that, in fact, the more aggression an individual used the more he wanted to use. After watching violent acts even those who did not commit a violent act themselves were desensitized to the degree of violence used by others and less sympathetic towards the victims (Thomas *et al.* 1977).

Of course, aggression that is expressed creatively (rechannelled or sublimated) is usually well rewarded. Sarcasm, for example, may be looked upon not only as a form of verbal aggression but also as cleverness. Being aggressively competitive may result in gaining a first prize.

It is important at this stage to establish the difference between aggressive behaviour and assertive behaviour. Assertiveness is sometimes referred to as emotional freedom and means that one can disagree, say no, point out things one does not like and generally express what one feels: however, it is not intended to hurt or destroy and does not involve the use of physical violence.

Case History

Mr Wychowski brought his daughter who had cut her hand to the accident and emergency department. The accident happened when she put her hand through the new patio window while playing tennis with a friend, although both girls had been warned not to play near the window. Mr Wychowski had come home from work at 6 p.m. after a really heavy day at the office, through a long traffic jam, to be greeted by his wife in a very distressed state and a crying child. His wife was very angry and upset particularly since she had repeatedly suggested that the window should be made of safety glass but he had preferred to cut the cost by using less expensive materials.

He arrived in accident and emergency with his daughter and because he had had no previous experience of such a department he simply sat down with his child in a row with others: there was no receptionist at the desk at the time. His daughter's hand was not bleeding now but he felt it needed to be looked at just the same. After a while he asked a fellow casualty if there was anything he should do since he was unfamiliar with the routine. The fellow casualty assumed that someone had taken his particulars and replied: 'No—you just sit and wait. They'll call you when they want you.' A receptionist arrived at the desk but he assumed she would call him when she wanted him and, anyway, he did not like to get up and go over to her since it would have looked as if he was blatantly disregarding the information given by his fellow casualty who was still sitting next to him.

He sat for nearly an hour while other people got up and went into cubicles. He then went up to the desk (his fellow casualty having gone into a cubicle himself) and said that he had been there for an hour or more. The receptionist replied 'Did you book in?'. He replied, a little surprised, 'Book in— no.' In a patronizing tone she pointed out: 'Well, we're not telepathic, you know.' He apologized and gave the details she asked for before returning to his seat to wait for another half an hour. A couple of urgent casualties were rushed in and there was great activity. After another half an hour he told his daughter to sit there while he went to phone his wife. The telephone was out of order. While he was away the daughter's name was called but at 10 years old she was unused to hearing herself called 'Miss' and instead of pronouncing her surname 'Wychowski' the nurse called 'Miss Wychi'. By the time he got back his little girl was quite distressed because the man now sitting next to her was vomiting into a bowl. They moved to another seat where they sat for a further half an hour. Meanwhile, two nurses went into a room to have their break and could be seen through the door laughing and joking with a porter over a cup of coffee for 20 minutes. Mr Wychowski stopped a student nurse and said, 'I've been here over two hours now—when am I likely to be seen, my daughter's cut her hand?' She told him they were very busy tonight and that everyone was having a long wait and walked away with a pleasant smile. After another 20 minutes Mr Wychowski saw two other nurses go into the little room for their break. Things seemed to have calmed down and another nurse was standing talking to a porter in the corner. A man and woman in white coats left the department laughing loudly. 'Look,' said Mr Wychowski to the next nurse he happened to see, 'I've been here hours; when will I be seen?' She told him that the doctors had just gone for their supper break and he would be seen when they got back. He asked if there was anywhere he could get something to eat and was told that there was a drinks machine but that it was usually out of order.

The doctors returned 25 minutes later. This time the girl's father took her by the hand into the cubicle into which the male doctor had just gone. Sister and staff nurse were fooling around with a piece of sticky tape on the doctor's stethoscope. Sister looked up in surprise and asked 'Can I help you?' Her tone was rather authoritarian. 'I've been here since bloody six this evening, it's about bloody time you did your job and saw this child's hand.' At this, sister drew back the curtain and said, 'Will you wait outside please. You will be called as soon as your turn comes—we've been unusually busy tonight as you would know if you had been here since 6 p.m.' He retreated and sat back with the other casualties who were 'tut-tutting' about overworked nurses and inconsiderate patients who want to jump the queue.

Sister, however, realized that something was wrong if Mr Wychowski had been there for that length of time and sent the staff nurse to find out why. The daughter's notes could not be found because they had been placed incorrectly on the pile containing the notes of those patients who were to be followed up in other clinics. The receptionist called him up to the desk and asked him to give her his daughter's details. He explained very crossly that he had already done that but she told him that he had not given them to her since she had only recently come on duty. He repeated the information and sat down again. After 10 minutes he got up and marched his daughter into a cubicle, which had just been vacated. 'Right,' he said, 'you see her *now*.' Sister replied, 'We are going to if *you* will please sit down outside.' Sister took hold of the child's hand and added, 'You are only upsetting her in here. Wait outside please.' With this she put her hand on his arm and gently pushed him towards the curtain to go outside. He grabbed her arm and pushed her off his arm. 'Right — I don't have to take this, call the porter, nurse!' said Sister. The porter hurried in and took hold of Mr Wychowski's arm, pulling him gently towards the hallway. His daughter was screaming as Sister tried to keep her with her in the cubicle. It was then that Mr Wychowski took a swing at the porter and two policemen who had just brought in a drunk rushed to his aid.

EXERCISE 2

Imagine that you are the accident and emergency sister and in a few lines report the incident as she sees it.

EXERCISE 3

Write a few lines about this incident as if you were Mr Wychowski telling the tale.

EXERCISE 4

Compare the case history and the two accounts you have just written. What is the difference between subjective and objective reporting?

Case History

Martin was brought into the psychiatric unit by the police who had left him saying, 'They know how to deal with "nutters" like you here mate.' He had been placed on a section of the Mental Health Act 1983 and the nurse in charge had spent some time checking the papers and talking to the social worker involved. One of the nurses had felt it necessary to discuss the statement made by one of the police officers about 'nutters' with the constable, pointing out that it was an inappropriate word to use and quite offensive. The exchange had been pleasant and they had shaken hands as he left and both were smiling.

Martin was taken, smelling strongly of alcohol, to a side room and asked if he would like a cup of tea. He told the nurse that he had not eaten since early morning and was very hungry. She told him 'There'll be a meal soon' and left, leaving his room door open. After 10 minutes' wait he decided he would come out and look for his cup of tea or some food—perhaps she had meant him to do that anyway and would be wondering why he was still in the room. He was far from disturbed at that time and, in fact, he was quite calm once the police had left. He could not see the nurse because she had gone off the ward in pursuit of another patient who was continually disappearing. What he had found though was the kitchen. Once inside, he saw a sandwich, picked it up and began to eat it. 'Get your bloody hands off that,' bellowed a voice from the doorway. He put the sandwich down and said how sorry he was but the other patient just grabbed the sandwich, looked at the bitten piece and threw it in the rubbish bin before storming out. The ward domestic, having heard the shouting, came into the kitchen and ordered Martin out. He went into the dayroom and sat down, unfortunately, next to a man who at that time was mute. Martin asked him what he ought to do but he did not answer. He asked the patient opposite but she, being deaf, just smiled at him then roared with laughter. The nurse who had promised the tea came into the dayroom looking flustered. 'John,' she said looking at Martin. 'I told you to stay in your room—I've made you a cup of tea and it's sitting there getting cold.' He got up and went out with her. 'I thought you'd forgotten,' he said. 'We're very busy you know—you're not the only one of 30 patients who needs help,' she replied. She was actually feeling rather bad since it had dawned on her how dangerous it could have been leaving this patient alone as she had done—but what could she do when she had seen Mrs Grant running off like that and no other nurse around? The charge nurse came into the sideroom. Martin stopped drinking his tea and looked at it very suspiciously. 'What's in it, then?' he asked staring at the cup. 'Oh my God,' replied the charge nurse, 'not another one today who realizes I am chucking my career away just to poison him.' Both nurses laughed but Martin did not. The nurse in charge approached him rapidly and put his arm around Martin's shoulder in a friendly gesture. The other nurse closed the door since she did not want other patients listening to the conversation. Martin backed off, saying 'Keep your hands off— I know what's going on.' The nurse reopened the door a little and called, 'David, can you join us for a minute?' Staff Nurse David came in and took his spectacles off, placing them in his pocket. 'I'm warning you lot,' Martin said. 'I'll kill the lot of you. Where I come from it's survival of the fittest. I'm not afraid of you nor the pigs that brought me here.'

At this point another man came in and said to the charge nurse, 'I can't see him while he's like this. I'll prescribe something,' and then left. The charge nurse told Martin to undress and that he would give him something to help him relax and reassured him that nobody would hurt him. He approached him again and once more Martin backed off. The other two nurses came forward slightly and at this Martin backed off again but this time he was against the wall. Suddenly he kicked out and punched the nearest nurse. Suddenly *he* was on the floor and the room seemed full of people, most of whom were on top of him.

EXERCISE 5

Rewrite this passage but interpret each thing that happens and each statement as if you were Martin. Try to envisage what he feels like during the episode.

EXERCISE 6

Here is a list of some of the factors that contribute to an aggressive incident. When you have read the two case histories related above, indicate whether each factor applied to Mr Wychowski or Martin, or to both. If YES, please tick. If NO, leave a blank.

Mr Wychowski   Martin

1 *Communication difficulties*
Was either of them misunderstood; did people fail to listen to them; did anyone patronize or belittle them or was anyone rude?

2 *Waiting*
Was either of them kept waiting, especially if it was for a long time and particularly if nobody really seemed to care?

3 *Restrictions*
Were there any rules or regulations which were frustrating? Did either of them have to go 'through the proper channels' or comply with bureaucracy?

4 *Overcrowding/space limitations*
Did either of them have to remain in one area for any length of time, especially if they did not want to be there? Did they have to be with people they would not have chosen to be with?

5 *Fear/uncertainty regarding the future*
Was either of them frightened and, if so, of what? Did either of them have any real cause for anxiety over their future safety/freedom?

6 *Feeling responsible for another person's safety*
Did either of them feel the need to act as advocate for another, particularly if this individual was more vulnerable than he was? Did either of them feel guilty about what had happened to someone else?

7 *Personality clashes and dominance rivalry*
Do you think that Mr Wychowski or Martin was at any time in a win-or-lose situation which could have involved loss of face? Was there a situation in which someone else was ignoring something they had said?

8 *Feeling unaccepted or neglected*
Was there a time when one of them might have felt that other people were getting better treatment?

9 *Inability to control behaviour in the way one usually does*
Is there any evidence of a loss of inhibition on either client's part, e.g. did either have brain damage or had either been drinking alcohol or taking drugs? Even being tired and hungry can lead to difficulty in controlling one's temper.

10 *Psychiatric disorders*
Some psychiatric disorders result in the client's seeing something very frightening that nobody else can see (hallucination) and believing people are going to harm them (delusion). Do either of these apply?

11 *Violence as a way of life*
Do either Mr Wychowski or Martin habitually use violence?

12 *Violence as a subcultural norm or a temporary norm*
Do you know if either man comes from an area where there is a lot of violence continually? Was the general atmosphere in A & E that day a very violent one?

13 *Not being able to do what one is asked to do*
Was either of the men frustrated at not being able to do something because of a personal weakness or lack of understanding?

continued on next page

continued

Mr Wychowski   Martin

14 *In self-defence*
   Did Mr Wychowski or Martin feel that they needed to defend themselves
   against a real or imagined threat?
15 *Rewards for violence*
   Refer back to the beginning of the chapter and consider instrumental
   violence. Was instrumental violence a factor in the behaviour of either
   man?

Prevention and Management of Aggressive Behaviour

The key to management is, of course, that prevention is better than having to deal with
an incident of physical aggression. In both the case histories a number of things could
have been done to reduce the likelihood of aggression. If we take the example of Mr
Wychowski, it is possible to see how simple things like manipulation of the environment
could have helped. For example, there could have been a notice telling people what to
do when they arrive in the accident and emergency department which would have helped to
prevent tension, as would a system for indicating how long casualties would have to wait for
attention — perhaps by giving each casualty a numbered disk when he arrives and displaying
prominently the number of the person currently being attended to. The reception area
could have been made more pleasant by providing magazines, newspapers, and even a
video or television, as long as there was enough space to ensure that people were able to
avoid having to look at it if they did not wish to do so. Chairs could have been more
informally grouped because sitting in rows allows little choice of who may be beside, in
front of or behind one. Tea and coffee facilities should be available, although there should
be a notice warning of the hazards of giving fluids to a casualty without first consulting
a nurse. Children regularly use accident and emergency departments and although children
who are injured may not want to play, their accompanying brothers and sisters will be
restless unless toys are available. It is quite calming to sit and watch brightly-coloured
tropical fish swimming in a tank.

The next group of contributory factors is that concerned with communication. The
attitude of the staff, and the manner in which they spoke to Mr Wychowski, left a lot
to be desired. It should be remembered that to Mr Wychowski the most important person
in the department that night was his daughter. Even though her injury was a minor one
it would have helped if someone had shown some interest in it. Perhaps it could have been
dealt with at home if his wife had not been so upset and so angry with him about using
cheap glass, but the fact remains that he had come to a hospital. Although we have to
assume that the nurses had assessed from a distance that there was no urgency, it would
have helped him if they had set his mind at rest on this point. He would certainly agree
that nurses need to have a break but it is difficult to have to watch someone doing nothing
for 20 minutes when she had just said that the department was very busy that night: perhaps
she might have been a little more discreet and shut the door.

EXERCISE 7

> How might the incident in the psychiatric department have been prevented?

If prevention fails or the incident could not have been prevented, there are twenty rules to be remembered:

1 If physically threatened, try to stay calm and, if you can, sit down and invite the other person to talk it over.
2 Appreciate their feelings and tell them you can see and understand how angry they are and why. This may make further violence unnecessary.
3 If alone, always try to get out of the situation or summon help.
4 Do not all talk at once. Let the person who has the best relationship with the aggressive individual do the talking in a calm manner.
5 Use the person's name.
6 Use the least possible force and never continue to use restraint when it is no longer necessary since this makes the assailant more angry.
7 Work as a team—if you have time, make a very quick plan.
8 Be firm in manner and firm in restraint.
9 Hold large joints in a way that reduces leverage.
10 If a weapon is involved use something to block it. Put something between you and the weapon.
11 The floor is one of the safest places on which to restrain a person, for he cannot fall and nor can you; it also reduces leverage.
12 If you can, remove his shoes—this will make a kick less painful—but obviously this will only be necessary if he continues to struggle. It is wise for nurses never to wear anything which could injure a patient, or themselves, such as elaborate earrings, wristwatches or brooches.
13 Try to have material between your hands and his skin since it reduces bruising. A blanket rolled across the patient's body and held down at the sides is a useful restraint if he is very disturbed and continues to struggle.
14 Make sure that the assailant can breathe whatever position he is in. Keep an eye on his face.
15 Be sensitive to when he ceases to fight and struggle, and show him verbally and physically that it is all over.
16 Make sure someone stays with them after the incident but ensure that there is support readily available for that person just in case the situation flares up again.
17 Try not to lose your temper because if you do you may lose control and will regret it if you hurt someone more than was necessary just because your restraint got out of control.
18 Remember that others who witness the incident will probably find it terrifying. As soon as possible spare some time for the witnesses.

19 Once the incident is over and you have some time, sit down and look at why it happened. Look at the action that was taken to deal with it: we learn from our mistakes.
20 Do not forget that the incident happened but do not also hold it against the client for ever and, as a consequence, keep reminding him of it.

NB Every health authority should have its own policy for the management of aggressive incidents and it is important to familiarize yourself with this.

SELF-EVALUATION

1 List as many theories as you can relating to why man becomes aggressive.
2 There are two types of aggressive behaviour. One is called hostile aggression but what is the other?
3 Give an example of the type of aggression you have just named, explaining how it differs from hostile aggression.
4 Some people believe that if you watch aggression on television it will reduce your own drive towards aggression. This is referred to as _____ satisfaction.
5 Aggression which is used in order to protect the underdog is referred to as _____ aggression.
6 Use of the mental defence mechanism of sublimation may result in aggression being expressed in what form?
7 Identify six reasons why aggressive behaviour may occur in the crowd watching a football match.
8 What is the difference between aggressive behaviour and assertive behaviour?

Answers will be found on p. 92, except those for Question 1 which are given in the text.

REFERENCES

Bandura, A. (1973) *Aggression: A Social Learning Analysis.* Englewood Cliffs NJ: Prentice-Hall, 325–345.
Dollard, J. Doob, I. W., Miller, N. E., Mowrer, O. H. & Sears, R. R. (1939) *Frustration and Aggression.* New Haven, Conn: Yale University Press, 322.
Geen, R. G. & Quanty, M. B. (1977) The catharsis of aggression. In Berkowitz L. (ed.) *Advances in Experimental Social Psychology*, Vol 10. New York: Academic Press, 328.
Owen, D. R. (1973) The 47 XYY male. *Psychology Review*, **78**, 209–233, 55.
Patterson, G. R., Littman, R. A. & Bricker, W. A. (1967) Assertive behaviour in children. A step towards a theory of aggression. *Monographs of the Society of Research in Child Development*, Serial No 113, **32(5)**, 327.

Steuer, F. B., Applefield, J. M. & Smith, R. (1971) Televised aggression and the interpersonal aggression of preschool children. *Journal of Experimental Child Psychology*, **11**, 442–447, 328.
Thomas, M. H., Horton, R. W., Lippincott, E. C. & Drabman, R. S. (1977) Destination to portrayals of real-life aggression as a function of exposure to television violence. *Journal of Personality and Social Psychology*, **35**, 450–458, 330.

FURTHER READING

Atkinson, R. L., Atkinson, R. C. & Hilgard, E. R. (1983) *Introduction to Psychology*. New York: Harcourt Brace Jovanovich.
Cardwell, S. (1984) Violence in accident and emergency departments. *Nursing Times*, 4 April.
Howie, C. (1985) Violence—the enemy within. *Nursing Times*, 17 April.
Vousden, M. (ed.) (1987) Control of aggressive patients. *Nursing Times*, 1 July, 28.

Chapter 10

The Patient with a Sexual Problem

Sexuality refers to the way in which we demonstrate our maleness or femaleness. We are born, having been influenced by chromosomes and hormones around the 12th week of life in the uterus, as biologically male or female and through the process of our upbringing we take on the behaviour which our society deems appropriate for that role (Fling & Manosevitz 1972). Freud developed a complicated theory about how children in the phallic stage of psychosexual development (3–6 years) copy the parent of the same sex because of the love and wish to possess the parent of the opposite sex, but the analytical aspects of what goes on at this age have, of late, been queried. Certainly, children imitate adult behaviour and by the age of three can distinguish male from female (Maccoby & Jacklin 1975). Before this age there is very little difference in a child's behaviour whether it is male or female. Margaret Mead (1935), having studied three tribes in New Guinea, showed that there is no universally accepted female or male behaviour. In one tribe men and women were equal and shared all aspects of work but both sexes avoided aggressive behaviour; in another tribe both men and women were equally aggressive and had no apparent maternal or nurturing instincts, and in the third the women were physically stronger because they did all the physical work, hunted, defended, and so on, while the men cooked, painted, danced and generally made themselves acceptable to their womenfolk. However, in each culture the characteristics that it deems appropriate will be rewarded: for example, Broverman *et al.* (1970) demonstrated that the mentally healthy male was said to be aggressive, independent, objective and the female submissive, dependent, subjective and suggestible. Bem (1975) believes that a healthy state is when there is psychological androgyny: in other words, we have both male and female stereotyped behaviours within the one individual. So it would be acceptable for men to be gentle and passive and for women to be assertive and achievement-oriented at appropriate times. In fact, the work of Wolfish & Myerson (1980), Radlove (1984), and Baucom & Aiken (1984) revealed that androgynous women were happier with their own sexuality and had more frequent orgasms than stereotypically feminine women and that androgynous couples seemed to be more satisfied with their life together.

SEXUAL DYSFUNCTION

Much sexual dysfunction in females appears to stem from the general inhibition and coyness which is regarded as a feminine characteristic, and in males from the need to be always interested in sex, always dominant and never failing (Jehu 1979; Stock 1984). Many difficulties stem from anxieties about pregnancy, physical damage and ignorance, from couples failing to communicate with each other, particularly about their sexual likes and dislikes, and as a consequence of marital disharmony, for when the relationship is poor it often follows that the sexual side of the marriage is also poor. It is important to try to establish the cause: it is usually one of the psychological problems mentioned above and very rarely physical. Drugs, particularly antihypertensives, psychotropic agents, anticholinergics and opiates may result in dysfunction, as may certain illnesses such as diabetes, multiple sclerosis and alcoholism which affect sex hormone levels. A localized infection can sometimes cause the problem, as can, very rarely, a malformation of the sexual organs.

Sexual intercourse has four stages:

Excitement phase: There is physiological and psychological arousal from stimulation of parts of the body which are termed erogenous zones (places which we like to have touched, kissed, bitten, and so on) and an increase in muscle tension, heart rate, blood pressure and respiration. In the female the vagina lubricates, and in the male erection occurs.

Plateau phase: The vaginal opening reduces in size, squeezing the penis and the glans penis swells inside the vagina. The penis is thrust up and down inside the vagina.

Orgasmic phase: Strong rhythmic contractions accompanied by ejaculation take place in the penis, and the walls of the vagina contract rhythmically.

Phase of resolution: The male needs a varying period of time before intercourse can take place again but the female, although she may be pleasantly exhausted, could physiologically have intercourse again straight away.

Dysfunction may occur at any stage throughout these phases and includes:

Frigidity: Reduced sexual arousal in the female. Occasionally primary, but more often secondary.

Vaginismus: Tightening of the vaginal muscles making intercourse impossible or painful.

Anorgasmia: Failure to achieve an orgasm. (Many women find that it is necessary for the clitoris to be stimulated during intercourse in order to achieve an orgasm and there is certainly nothing wrong with them if this is the case.)

Impotence: Failure to achieve or maintain an erection. Occasionally primary but more often secondary; sometimes with secondary impotence there is arousal failure or lack of desire. Primary impotence implies that an erection has never been achieved and secondary that erections have been maintained in the past.

Premature ejaculation: Ejaculation prior to entering the phase of orgasm.

Retarded ejaculation: Although this might seem a desirable state it is, in fact, very unfulfilling and may be non-ejaculation.

PREFERENCE DIFFERENCES

When we refer to someone's sexual orientation it means the direction or object of his or her desire. The majority of people are oriented towards members of the opposite sex (heterosexual) but a preference difference (in the past called a deviation) means that the individual is oriented towards something other than the normal, i.e. heterosexual, or is oriented towards a practice that is not regarded as being normal.

Homosexuality and lesbianism: Orientation towards members of the same sex.
Bestiality: Orientation towards sexual fulfilment with animals.
Necrophilia: Orientation towards sexual fulfilment with dead bodies.
Paedophilia: Orientation towards sexual fulfilment with children.
Transvestism: Orientation towards sexual fulfilment through dressing in the clothing of the opposite sex.
Fetishism: Orientation towards sexual fulfilment through being in contact with articles not usually associated with sexual fulfilment, e.g. leather, womens' undergarments.
Masochism and sadism: Orientation towards sexual fulfilment through receiving and giving pain.
Voyeurism: Orientation towards sexual fulfilment through observing others either in a state of undress or when making love.
Exhibitionism: Orientation towards sexual fulfilment through exhibiting the genitalia.
Frotteurism: Orientation towards sexual fulfilment through touching others, usually by pressing the genitalia against the person.
Transexuality: A feeling that one is biologically and genitally of one sex but psychologically of the opposite sex.

Case History

John was slow at school and left with no qualifications. His IQ as said to be dull–normal. He was unemployed and had married Maria, whom he met at a dance. The marriage was unsuccessful from the beginning and people blamed this on the fact that the couple had only known each other for two months before marrying. Maria found the sexual side of their marriage to be very unfulfilling and, when they were out together with friends or in the pub, would joke about John's inability to satisfy her. He tried just about everything in order to achieve what she wanted but she ridiculed all his efforts. He remembered his mother complaining about his father but describing him as an animal who saw sex as something one just did rather than something that was linked with love. He did not like his father very much and got on much better with his mother.

After a blazing row with his wife he left the home and went for a long walk which took him past some woodland. He said he got the urge to masturbate and went into the woods. He heard the sound of footsteps and realized that someone was coming along the footpath beside the wood. He knew by the sound that it was a woman. On impulse he moved to the edge of the wood and made a noise so that she would look in his direction. She was both shocked and scared and he remembered being pleased that she was both of these things, it giving him a feeling of power and success. He repeated this behaviour occasionally from then on, particularly when things were going badly at home. His wife's comments did not seem to matter so much anymore. He did not see it as a really dangerous piece of behaviour or harmful in any way because he knew he had no intention of hurting the women. Then, one day, a woman came along and instead of the usual reaction she was very angry, shouted at him, called him names and started towards him. He felt very angry, and at the same time, frightened.

The next day, he went into a park and hid near a place where he knew that children played. He saw a group of little girls playing ball and masturbated until they came fairly near to him. He put his hands in his pockets to pull his coat across in front of him and walked close to them: he called one of the little girls over and then exposed himself to her. She just stared at him and did not move, whereupon he impulsively grabbed her hand and placed it on his erect penis. He immediately ejaculated but suddenly realized that a park-keeper was running towards him. Before he could get away the keeper had grabbed him and was calling him all the names under the sun. The man was much stronger than him and was soon aided by a man walking his dog.

John was arrested and convicted. A psychiatrist recommended that he should receive psychiatric help. He was placed on a section of the Mental Health Act 1983 which allowed him to be detained compulsorily in a psychiatric unit for assessment and treatment.

John's treatment consisted of counselling him about his relationships with women, his feelings about his father, mother and wife, and his feelings about the situation which had resulted in his conviction. He was able to see how distressing it had been for his victims but he said the urge to do it had been overpowering. He was taught to relax and to try to use this technique whenever he felt anxious and at times when he might previously have felt the urge to expose himself. Through visual imagery he was helped to recreate scenes which would have resulted in an episode of his previous behaviour but this time to try to visualize alternative courses of action. It was necessary to develop his social skills and this was achieved through group work and role play. He particularly needed to become more assertive and express his wishes through words. He began to find that he was less tense, could visualize situations where he would now handle things differently and to speak up for himself more. It was not considered necessary to think of drugs which might suppress his sexual urges and he was only prescribed a small dose of tranquillizer to help him reduce his tension. By attending group therapy he was able to let others know why he was in hospital and to cope with his feelings of guilt and disgust.

His wife never visited him and he was later divorced: his father refused to see him but his mother visited occasionally. He worked with a female nurse on his problems with women and developed a close relationship with a female patient.

EXERCISE 1

List below the characteristics, interests and jobs that you think our society considers to be typically female or typically male.

Male	Female
1	
2	
3	
4	
5	
6	
7	
8	
9	
10	

continued on next page

continued

Having compiled this list try to rate yourself on a 1 (low correlation) to 10 (high correlation) scale. If, for example, you had described gentleness as a female characteristic, or interest in appearance as a feminine interest, decide how gentle or interested you are and give it a score. How androgynous are you?

EXERCISE 2

Design, in the spaces provided below, your own personal example of a sexually attractive man and woman. If you are female, design the male first and then try to envisage a sterotypical, sexually attractive female, and vice versa if you are male. Imagine that you are judging them in swimwear.

Male	*Female*
Height	. . . .
Hair	. . . .
Eyes	. . . .
Skin	. . . .
Mouth	. . . .
Teeth	. . . .
Ears	. . . .
Nose	. . . .
Neck	. . . .
Shoulders	. . . .
Chest	. . . .
Waist	. . . .
Weight	. . . .
General shape	. . . .
Hips	. . . .
Bottom	. . . .
Legs	. . . .
Feet	. . . .
Hands	. . . .

EXERCISE 3

Our body image is an internalized picture of what we think we look like. List below the ways in which someone's body image could be altered through ageing, illness, surgery or accident.

REFERENCES

Baucom, D. & Aitken, P. (1984) Sex role identity, marital satisfaction and response to behavioural marital therapy. *Journal of Consulting and Clinical Psychology*, **52**, 438–444.

Bem, S. (1975) Sex role adaptability: one consequence of psychological androgyny. *Journal of Consulting and Clinical Psychology*, **45**, 196–205.

Broverman, I., Broverman, D., Clarkson, F., Rosenkrantz, P. & Vogel, S. (1970) Sex role stereotypes and clinical judgements in mental health. *Journal of Consulting and Clinical Psychology*, **34**, 1–7.

Fling, S. & Manosevitz, M. (1972) Sex typing in nursery school children's play interests. *Developmental Psychology*, **7**, 146–152.

Jehu, D. (1979) *Sexual Dysfunction: A Behavioural Approach to Causation, Assessment and Treatment*. New York: John Wiley & Sons.

Maccoby, E. & Jacklin, C. (1975) *The Psychology of Sex Differences*. London: Oxford University Press.

Mead, M. (1935) *Sex and Temperament in Three Primitive Societies*. New York: Morrow & Co.

Radlove, S. (1984) Sexual response and gender roles. In Allgeier, E. & McCormick, N. (eds) *Changing Behaviour*. Palo Alto: Mayfield.

Stock (1984) Sex roles and sexual dysfunction. In Widon, C. (ed.) *Sex Roles and Psychopathology*. New York: Plenum Press.

Wolfish, S. & Myerson, M. (1980) Sex role identity and attitudes towards sexuality. *Archives of Sexual Behaviour*, **9**, 199–203.

FURTHER READING

Freedman, G. (1983) *Sexual Medicine*. Edinburgh: Churchill Livingstone.

Hargreaves, D. & Colley, A. (eds) (1986) *The Psychology of Sex Roles*. New York: Harper & Row.

Webb, C. (1985) *Sexuality, Nursing and Health*. Chichester: John Wiley & Sons.

Chapter 11

When Social Integration is a Problem

Case History

Name: Steven Castelloni
Age: 48 years
Religion: R/C
Marital status: divorced
Children: one son
Previous occupation: labourer
Contact with family: father visits about twice a year. No other contacts.
Date of admission: 1970 (at 31 years of age)

Admitted after an episode of violence towards his father. He claimed that everyone was against him and trying to get rid of him. Steven had been increasingly distant over a three-year period and the relationship with his wife had deteriorated. The relationship worsened after the birth of his son. His wife and mother-in-law had refused to allow Steven even to hold his child, saying that he was not a fit person to do so. Eventually they locked him out (he shared the house with his mother-in-law, in whose name it was). This practice of locking him out increased in frequency and he slept rough from time to time. He returned to his parents home and from there was seen by his general practitioner, who found him 'uncommunicative and bizarre in behaviour'. He was admitted to hospital from then on for periods ranging from three weeks to six months. His intelligence level was described as dull–average but he was barely literate, seemingly as the result of his constant truanting from school. His last admission was in 1976, and after six months in the admission ward he was transferred to a continuing-care area where he has remained ever since.

Current Behaviour (baseline)

Shows no interest in anything except smoking. Spends the day slouched in a chair, only getting up for meals or to wander aimlessly around the ward or hospital corridors. Retires to bed as early as he can. Looks unkempt, wearing his clothes in a careless manner and is reluctant to attend to hygiene or to shave. In fact, he lacks drive to do anything. He communicates only when it is essential to do so and appears to have no friends in the ward and no attachment to anything or anyone. In fact, he appears

76

to be unaware of those around him. He stares blankly downwards, seems to have lost all interest in reality, needs continual prompting by staff, maintains the same routine day after day and dislikes change.

Understanding Steven's Behaviour

Motivation can be defined very simplistically as 'the reasons why we do what we do'. Usually we do something in order to meet our own or others needs. Motivation may be conscious ('I did it because of A, B and C') or unconscious (a reason which is completely or partially hidden from us). It might appear that our motivation for becoming a nurse, for example, was to help others but it could be that it was a reasonably secure job or it paid better than others we could get at the time. Maybe it gave a certain status which, perhaps, we knew would please our parents. It is very unusual for someone to say at interview that she wants to become a nurse for the power that she will have over others!

EXERCISE 1

To each of the following questions make an instant response. When you have done that, sit and think of other reasons why you do that particular thing and list those also.
1 Why do you make yourself look presentable when you go to work?
2 Why do you change your bed sheets?

EXERCISE 2

Try to think as if you were Steven: answer the following questions from his point of view.
1 What kind of job do you think you could get outside hospital?
2 Where do you think you will live for the next ten years?
3 How do you see your future?
4 Why do you become anxious when any changes are proposed?

EXERCISE 3

Once again, try to put yourself in Steven's place and answer the following questions as you think he would.

1 Why don't you do the following things for yourself:
   (a) cook meals?
   (b) change your bed sheets without being told to?
2 Why don't you take care not to burn holes in your clothes when you smoke?
3 Why don't you keep yourself looking presentable?
4 Why don't you enter into conversation with others?
5 Why don't you look around at your environment and others in it?
6 Who depends on you?
7 To whom do you think you are important, and for what reason?
8 What successes have you had during the past year?
9 What do you think you can do well?
10 What gives you pleasure?
11 Why don't you make friends?
12 In one sentence explain how you feel about yourself and your life and future.

When you have completed this exercise you should have some insight into why Steven lacks motivation and why he does not mix with others.

EXERCISE 4

In order to motivate Steven it is important to take action to reverse some of the reasons you may have given in the above exercise. For example, you may have said in reply to Question 3 that:
   (a) nobody cares what I look like,
   (b) the clothes I am given are not mine, I didn't choose them and they are tatty anyway,
   (c) I have poor eyesight or coordination (as a result of medication) and therefore I cannot do up buttons, zips, etc,
   (d) everyone else looks just the same as I do,
   (e) if I look smart people might start showing an interest in me or they might think I'm getting better and try to discharge me.

It is possible to take action regarding these statements. For example, test his eyesight, praise him when he looks nice, let him choose new clothes that are his own. Try coming up with possible ways of working on the reasons you have given in response to Questions 1–12 of Exercise 3.

Socializing Steven

Wing & Brown (1970) identified a relationship between the poverty of the environment and the deterioration of the patient. They found that if his physical environment is improved, even if nothing else is improved, there will be an improvement in the patient's state, or the degree of 'clinical poverty' as it is called. They also discovered that if a patient does nothing he will deteriorate mentally more rapidly than would otherwise be the case and that the number of hours spent each day doing nothing is related to the degree of deterioration. First, we shall improve Steven's environment, making it brighter and more homely, with seating arrangements conducive to conversation, and so on. Coffee-table gatherings, interesting pictures on the walls, a full-length mirror, different curtains in different rooms, carpets and screened-off areas, particularly in the dormitory, should be provided. The level of interest shown by staff is an important motivating factor and if staff appear bright, interested and polite they set a good role-model. In the early stages it might be useful if only one or two nurses attempt to make the initial relationship with Steven. It will take time to develop a rewarding relationship since he is likely to be suspicious and resistant to the process. Once a relationship had been established, one of these nurses might accompany him to social gatherings but simply allow him to go in and stay for a few minutes and then leave if he wishes. Through the relationship he might be encouraged to help with a little part of the arrangements for some social activity on the ward such as an afternoon cup of tea with three or four of the residents. Gradually, more people can be introduced into his circle of acquaintances and group activities undertaken, such as walks or shopping trips. Eventually, a small group of residents might be encouraged to develop and practise very simple social skills, gradually working up to more complex ones through role-play. Alternatively, a token economy scheme (another technique of behaviour modification) could be used whereby Steven is given tokens in exchange for demonstrating desirable social behaviour; he can exchange the tokens for sweets or other goods at a later date. Any efforts made by Steven should be rewarded with praise or other positive responses. As Wing & Freudenberg (1961) showed, a nurse who is stimulated and interested can do a lot to improve the functioning of even the most severely ill, chronic patient.

EXERCISE 5

Look back at your answers to Exercises 1, 2, 3 and 4. In the future it is hoped that patients will not remain in large institutions for long periods of time—how could you ensure that a newly-admitted patient does not end up in a similar state to the one in which we find Steven?

THE INDIVIDUAL AT ODDS WITH SOCIETY

Psychopathy, or sociopathy as it is sometimes called, is a character disorder in which the individual demonstrates the personality traits, emotional responses and behaviour patterns listed below. Numerous theories have been propounded on why this disorder should develop, e.g. Sim (1974) who argues that there is an abnormal electroencephalogram pattern rather like that of a child, which might account for some of the childlike behaviour as opposed to mature adult activity. Bowlby's (1965) theory relates to early maternal deprivation leading to an inability to develop relationships, and failure to develop the super-ego or conscience because the mother is unable to instil a sense of right and wrong in her child. Cleckley (1967) believes that the psychopath actually does things in order to be punished because he likes it.

Cognitive Features

Poorly developed conscience
Little sense of responsibility
Thoughts of self predominate
Manipulative
Lying very convincingly
Does not seem to learn by past errors
Wants what he/she wants *now* and does not consider waiting or delaying gratification of urges.

Emotional Features

Feels little or no guilt, shame or remorse
Cannot empathize with others
Large amounts of self-pity
Unable to receive or give love

Behaviour

Selfish
Promiscuous
Impulsive
Charming
Destroys others around him/her

Using Henderson's (1939) classification, there are three types of psychopath:

1 The aggressive psychopath whose main feature is the impulsive and repetitive use of violence with no regard for his victim, in order to achieve his ends.
2 The inadequate psychopath, who lives a parasitic life, dependent on others, using them and manipulating their lives.
3 The creative psychopath—the typical 'con man' who uses his wits to deceive and cheat: charming until he has obtained what he wants, ruthless and totally selfish, and often very successful, like J. R. Ewing depicted in *Dallas*.

Case History: Thomas the Terrible

Thomas was first admitted to the psychiatric department having slashed his wrists following the break-up of his relationship with a married woman. His next admission was arranged through the courts after he had been involved in an assault on a woman he worked with. During a weekend leave he became drunk and smashed the windows of a neighbour's house because the neighbour would not let him use his telephone. He absconded twice and was referred back to the courts and sent to prison. He came out of prison six months later, having been a model inmate. He had four jobs in the space of a year, each ending in a violent argument with a superior. He overdosed after the loss of the last job, which coincided with a row with the women he was living with, during which he beat her up, necessitating several sutures in her face. During his stay in the department he always seemed to be present when there was trouble, never directly involved but on the fringe. He selected the most vulnerable patients, and to some extent the most vulnerable staff, and used them as a shoulder to cry on, telling them how badly people had treated him in the past. He was always in the wrong place at the wrong time, always saying that he had thought it was where someone had told him to be. According to him he was never to blame although he always got the blame. He borrowed cigarettes from those patients who wouldn't try to get them back and got other patients to do his share of the ward chores, saying that he wasn't up to it or that he knew he would only do them incorrectly and get told off yet again. They felt very sorry for him. He taunted another male patient until a violent scene erupted and then denied all responsibility, putting himself in the position of the innocent victim of a brutal, unwarranted attack. He also encouraged a married female patient to tell her husband she would be better off without him 'just to see his reaction', with devastating results for the woman and her husband.

EXERCISE 6

Having read through Thomas's history and the account of his period in an admission unit, try to identify those aspects of his behaviour that are particularly undesirable, using the following headings:

Aspects relating to his inability to respond to stress without violence.
Manipulative behaviour.
Self-destructive behaviour.

Taking each area in turn, what could be done to help Thomas to develop an alternative approach and how might staff mitigate the effect that Thomas had on the ward environment, staff and patients?

REFERENCES

Bowlby, J. (1965) *Child Care and the Growth of Love*. Harmondsworth: Penguin Books.
Cleckly, B. (1967) *The Mask of Sanity*. New York: Basic Books.
Sim, M. (1974) *Guide to Psychiatry*. Edinburgh: Churchill Livingstone.
Wing, J. K. & Brown, G. W. (1970) *Institutionalism and Schizophrenia*. Cambridge: Cambridge University Press.
Wing, J. K. & Freudenberg, R. K. (1961) The response of severely ill chronic schizophrenic patients to social stimulation. *American Journal of Psychiatry*, **118**, 311–322.

FURTHER READING

Stokes, G. and Keen, I. (1987) Developing self-care skills and reducing institutional behaviour in a long-stay psychiatric ward. *Journal of Advanced Nursing*, January, 35.

Watts, F. & Bennett (eds) (1983) *Theory and Practice of Psychiatric Rehabilitation*. Chichester: John Wiley.

Youth Development Trust Manchester (1983) *Reflected Images*. (Read 'Silent Protest' relating to what it feels like to 'be observed rather than understood'.)

Chapter 12

Therapy Options

There is a wide range of services designed to help those with mental health problems and their carers. The following figure may be looked upon as a flowchart and gives an idea of the settings in which care takes place, the personnel involved and the therapy options.

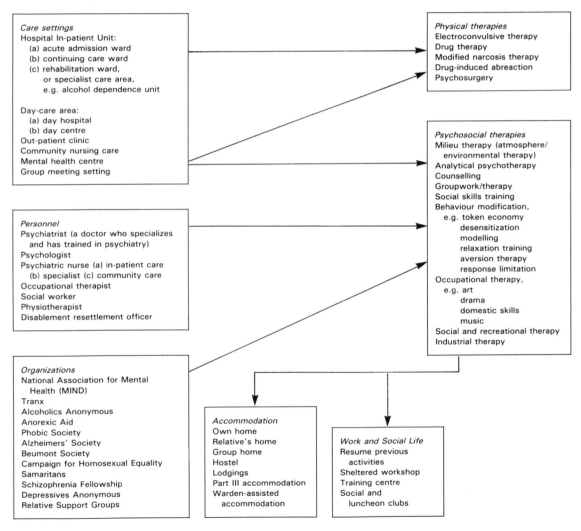

UNDERSTANDING PHYSICAL AND PSYCHOSOCIAL THERAPIES

Drug Therapy

The main groups of drugs used in psychiatry are as follows:

Major tranquillizers

Used to produce a calm state of mind and reduce psychotic symptoms without clouding of consciousness.

Examples: Chlorpromazine (Largactil), a phenothizine-group drug
        Haloperidol (Serenace), a butyrophenone-group drug

Major tranquillizers given in depot injection form

These injections may be given at weekly to monthly intervals. They avoid the necessity to remember to take oral medication since drug compliance is a major difficulty with some clients.

Examples: Flupenthixol decanoate (Depixol), a thioxanthene drug
        Haloperiodol (Haldol)

Minor tranquillizers

Used to relieve anxiety for periods of up to four months. Some patients have been prescribed these drugs for many years but they continue to take them more to avoid the unpleasant effects of ceasing to take them rather than to relieve anxiety. Sometimes called anxiolytics.

Examples: Diazepam (Valium)
        Chlordiazepoxide (Librium)

Sedatives/hypnotics

Non-barbiturate sedatives are used nowadays, usually to relieve insomnia, sometimes to prevent withdrawal symptoms.

Examples: Nitrazepam (Mogadon)
        Chlormethiazole (Heminevrin)

Antidepressants

(a) Monoamine oxidase inhibitors. Food substances containing tyramine should not be taken at the same time as these drugs, e.g. cheese, Bovril, pickled herrings.

(b) Tricyclics

Examples: MAOI group   Tranylcypromine (Parnate)
                        Phenelzine (Nardil)
        Tricyclic group   Amitriptyline (Tryptizol)
                        Imipramine (Tofranil)

Mood-stabilizing drugs

Used to relieve mood swings. The point between a therapeutic level in the body and a toxic level is small and it is essential, therefore, to ensure that regular serum levels are checked. Sometimes called normothymics.
Example: Lithium carbonate (Priadel; Camcolit)

EXERCISE 1

List in a column the drugs that you are currently administering which fall into the categories specified above. Alongside each drug write the initials of a patient who is receiving it and then try to establish exactly why the drug is being given to him. In a third column note any side-effects that you believe to be attributable to the patient's drug therapy.

Electroconvulsive Therapy (ECT)

ECT, or electroplexy as it is also known, is a treatment in which 200–400 milliamps of electric current at under 100 volts is passed through the brain of an anaesthetized patient for 0.3 of a second. The patient, who has also been given a muscle relaxant, may twitch or jerk a little. Following recovery from the anaesthetic he may experience a temporary disturbance of memory which lasts for an hour or so. This treatment, which under most circumstances requires the prior consent of the patient, is performed to influence mood, either to lift it if the patient is depressed or to lower it if he is manic.

EXERCISE 2

Identify a patient who is to receive ECT. Describe the preparation of the patient, both physical and psychological. Name the drugs which were used when ECT was given and the purpose of each drug. Describe the recovery period.

Modified Narcosis

Using hypnosedatives and major tranquillizers the patient is helped to sleep for 18 out of every 24 hours for about two weeks. During this time very skilful nursing care is required if the patient is to avoid the complications of prolonged bed rest.

Drug-induced Abreaction

The patient is given an intravenous anaesthetic, or ether administered on a mask, in order to encourage him to talk freely about his problems. Obviously, the drug is given very slowly since one does not want the patient to go to sleep but simply to remove some of his inhibitions and get him to talk.

Psychosurgery

Operations of this type on the brain are never carried out without the patient's informed consent. There are a number of slightly different operations but basically they are to relieve chronic anxiety, particularly when it occurs in someone whose premorbid personality was a 'good' one.

Psychosocial Therapies

Milieu Therapy

This is an atmosphere or an environment in which everything that goes on has a therapeutic intent. How residents are treated, who does what, how the rules are made and the relationships within the group sharing the environment are looked upon as being essential components of treatment.

Analytical psychotherapy

The psychotherapist, who is highly trained and has himself undergone some form of analysis, tries to discover the origins of the client's distress by focusing on things that he may have forgotten for one reason or another, particularly events which occurred during his childhood.

Counselling

Counselling is a way of helping people to identify, explore and understand their problems and, having looked at the options open to them, come to a decision as to what, if anything, they want to do about their situation. Through the skills of the counsellor the conversation becomes meaningful: such skills include the use of open questions rather than ones which require a 'yes' or 'no' answer, paraphrasing or putting into précis form what clients have said and checking that it is what they meant. One of the greatest skills is that of listening and allowing periods of silence, since these make space for clients to think.

Groupwork/therapy

A group of people meeting together may focus on a particular subject but many other things go on within that group setting which can be helpful to the individual: these other things are referred to as the group dynamics. In group therapy, people learn that they are not alone with their problems and gain hope since others have experienced the same problems and come through them. People learn from one another so that dependence on one person, i.e. the nurse or therapist, is minimised.

Social skills training

This kind of training uses the principles of behaviour modification (see below) and is usually carried out as groupwork with the focus on such things as asserting oneself, mixing in social situations, presenting oneself in a favourable light, and so on. The leader helps members to look at various strategies which may be useful in certain situations and, usually through role-play, gives them the opportunity to act out the situations and their new behaviour patterns again and again until they feel confident. Later, the work has to be translated into 'real-life' situations outside the group and this is usually achieved by giving homework, i.e. asking participants to try out in their 'real life' something that they have practised in the group and to report back during the next session.

Behaviour modification

Behaviour modification uses the principles of learning in order to help an individual to change some aspect of his behaviour which, usually, he has identified as being the cause of his problems. For example, it might be that he finds it difficult to travel by train, in which case the approach could be to use the technique of desensitization—this involves establishing a hierarchy of situations that would worry him, ranging from just thinking about travelling on a train through to being in an underground train which is stuck in a tunnel. The client is then taught to relax, and once he has mastered this technique he is helped to progress through the hierarchy of feared situations until he can conquer them.

Cognitive therapy may be incorporated in this treatment. Cognitive therapy involves helping the client to identify how his mood is linked to the way he thinks (cognition), to identify the irrational elements of his thinking and to look for a more constructive way of thinking. 'Modelling' will be incorporated since the therapist will be travelling with the client and will model or demonstrate how to stay calm and what to do in situations.

Token economy is a form of therapy in which desirable behaviour is encouraged by giving the client either a token resembling a poker chip, praise or some other reward such as privileges, in exchange for desirable elements of behaviour. A patient who has a problem in controlling his temper might be rewarded for each hour during which he expressed himself in an acceptable manner. The reward is referred to as positive reinforcement: it increases the likelihood of that particular behaviour being repeated.

Aversion therapy does the opposite and is used to discourage an undesirable behaviour such as drinking alcohol or dressing in the clothes of the opposite sex (transvestism) if it is identified as, and agreed to be, undesirable. It is achieved by coupling the activity which gives 'pleasure' with something that is unpleasant, such as feeling very ill or receiving pain. The usual method is to give drugs to produce the former and electric shocks for the latter.

Response limitation is a way of helping someone to control the behaviour which he wants to relinquish, for example, compulsive behaviour. The therapist establishes a baseline, i.e. how many times he performs the act, when, where and for how long: the therapist then agrees with the client a new pattern of behaviour which reduces the number of times that the act is carried out and the time during which it is done, for example, only washing his hands for five minutes instead of 20. Together they work gradually towards returning the client to his premorbid behaviour pattern.

Occupational, Social and Recreational and Industrial Therapies

Through art, drama and music people may be helped to express themselves and to achieve satisfaction. Every activity which is offered by an occupational therapy department in psychiatry has been analyzed and broken down into its various aspects, such as the degree of manual dexterity required, the amount of eye contact needed, the amount of cooperation versus competition, physical contact, concentration, and so on. Therefore, the therapy which best meets the patient's needs can be introduced. Social and recreational therapy helps people to make the most of leisure time, to integrate and achieve fulfilment through sedentary and physical activity. Industrial therapy tries to create as 'work-like' an environment as possible whilst appreciating the client's limitations, if any, at the time. Work forms an important part of the day for many people, giving order to the week, providing a sense of usefulness and fulfilment, giving them an opportunity to achieve, and providing companionship and a feeling of unity.

EXERCISE 3

Identify one or two of the patients you are working with by writing their initials on a sheet of paper. Beside their initials list those of the therapies described above that they are receiving and the purpose of the therapy in each individual's case. Once you have done this, identify the role of the nurse in each of these therapies.

FURTHER READING

Altschul, A. & McGovern, M. (1985) *Psychiatric Nursing*. Eastbourne: Baillière Tindall.
Bloor, M. (1986) 'Who'll make the tea?' *New Society* 31 January, 185–186.
Dally, P. & Connolly, J. (1981) *Physical Methods of Treatment in Psychiatry*. Edinburgh: Churchill Livingstone.
Longhorn, E. (1984) *Psychiatric Care and Conditions*. Chichester: John Wiley & Sons.
Simmons, S. & Brooker, C. (1986) *Community Psychiatric Nursing: A Social Perspective*. London: Heinemann.
Willson, Moya (1984) *Occupational Therapy in Short-term Psychiatry*. Edinburgh: Churchill, Livingstone.

Answers

Chapter 2 Self-evaluation

1 A dominant gene on an autosomal chromosome.
2 Each child has a 50/50 chance.
3 This refers to identical twins—genetically identical.
4 It provides a better opportunity for true assessment of genetic factors rather than nurture factors.
5 A chemical messenger released into the synapse. Dopamine. Noradrenaline. Acetylcholine.
6 Conflicting verbal and non-verbal messages, e.g. "I'm really interested", said while looking bored.
7 A person who was important to them had died when they were very young.
8 Lower, e.g. Class IV and V. Communication differences, readiness to diagnose or time allocation.
9 If you are told you are argumentative, you might argue against this. This ends up as proof that you *are* argumentative.
10 (a) Loss of prospects outside the institution. (b) More friends inside than out. (c) A readiness to come back to hospital willingly because it may hold out more for you than the community.

Chapter 3 Self-evaluation

1 If he is not unwilling to become an in-patient. This may mean that he accepts that he needs help but it is worthwhile to consider such possibilities as whether or not he actually realizes that he can refuse if he so wishes.
2 No. However, using common law principles the patient could be 'treated' in order to prevent physical damage to himself or another person. (Section 62 does not apply to informal patients.
3 Hormone implants and psychosurgery.
4 Yes. However, after he has been receiving this medication for a three-month period we would require either (a) his consent to continue treatment, or (b) a second opinion confirming its necessity.
5 Drugs (no second opinion is needed until a three-month period of drug treatment has elapsed) and electroconvulsive therapy.
6 No—not unless they are willing to come back.
7 Mental Health Review Tribunal.
8 Mental Health Act Commission.
9 Nearest relative or approved social worker, plus two doctors. A signature is also needed on behalf of the hospital managers (usually signed by the senior nurse on duty).

10 Place either on a section 5(4) by an RMN, if a doctor cannot be found quickly enough, or on a section 5(2) by the doctor: the former lasts for six hours and the latter for 72 hours.

Chapter 4   Self-evaluation

1   A phobia or a specific situation in which anxiety occurs.
2   Within the cerebrum. It gives rise to the emotional state.
3   Heart speeds up and its rate increases.
    Bronchioles dilate.
    Mouth dries (salivation reduced).
    Pupils dilate.
    Skin sweaty.
    Bladder muscle in the wall relaxes and the sphincter closes.
4   A means of protecting our mental state and self-image. It is also involved in helping us to present to the outside world the kind of picture of ourselves that we would wish them to see.
5   Loss of hearing—a person might not want to hear something which he believes is going to be said.
6   Hysterical dissociative state.
7   Chronic multiple physical symptoms with no physical origins or foundations.
8   In hospital addiction (Munchausen) syndrome the person consciously attempts to fake problems, as with the patient who places someone else's sputum in his own mouth in order to be able to expectorate it into his sputum pot in front of a nurse.
9   Limiting the number of times a person is able to carry out obsessive-compulsive behaviour.
10 (a) To answer this you should have considered the physical, psychological and social aspects of each family member's life and the total family life.
    (b) Check with the text of Chapter 4.

Chapter 5   Exercise 3: Helping James

1   Appropriate.
2   Inappropriate—he may drink them immediately and burn himself or he may simply push or throw them away, burning you.
3   Definitely inappropriate—he will put the others off their food in this state.
4   Inappropriate—nobody else will sleep.
5   Inappropriate—he is probably burning up a lot of energy anyway but it might be appropriate to let him 'jog' around the grounds (assuming you can keep up with him) if you think it would have a calming effect on him.
6   Inappropriate—if he smokes he probably needs to but do supervise him closely.
7   Inappropriate—the best way or deal with this is to say something like: 'It must be nice to feel like that, James.' It would not be appropriate to try to put him down in some way.
8   A very good intervention—he is suggestible and this does work.
9   Appropriate.
10 Inappropriate—tell him that you do understand and ask him to explain more clearly, refocusing him if necessary. Be prepared for him to be very irritated by your apparent stupidity.

11 Inappropriate—other patients may deal with what they see as an antisocial piece of behaviour in their own way! Explain the wisdom of privacy to James.
12 Inappropriate—far better to devise a way of encouraging him to use the toilet, e.g. a cigarette in there, or a magazine to look at.

Chapter 6 Self-evaluation—1

1 Alzheimer's disease, Pick's disease, Jacob-Creutzfeldt's disease, Huntington's chorea.
2 Jacob-Creutzfeldt's disease. Tissues and blood.
3 Through a dominant gene on an autosomal chromosome. 50:50 chance.
4 Shrunken, typical convoluted shape changed, ventricles enlarged, space between skull and brain increased.
5 In organic psychosis there is demonstrable cerebral pathology.
6 Apraxia—inability to carry out certain actions.
Agnosia—inability to recognize objects/find one's way around in familiar settings.
Confabulation—filling gaps in the memory with false information.
Echolalia—repeating the words of another person.
Choreo-athetoid movements—a combination of slow writhing movements and sudden jerky movements.

Chapter 6 Self-evaluation—2

1 Believing that one is dead.
2 A false sensory perception in the absence of an objective stimulus.
3 Olfactory (smell), optic (sight), tactile (touch), gustatory (taste) and auditory (hearing).
4 The sudden interruption of a flow of thought making it difficult or impossible for the person to continue with that line of thought.
5 Going round and round and never getting to the point.

Chapter 7 Exercise 2

1 False: 1 unit = 1 single whisky
1 sherry
1 glass wine
½ pint of beer
2 True.
3 True.
4 True.
5 True.
6 True.
7 False: it is a cerebral depressant and the apparent stimulant effect is due to the reduction in inhibitions.
8 False: mainlining refers to intravenous injection.

9 False: it is low in Moslem countries and high in France and Italy.

10 False: the method is just one of the dangers. The substances themselves are toxic.

Chapter 7   Exercise 3

1 Agitation, restlessness, tremor, flushing, sweating, delirium. Her slightly hostile approach towards questioning, and the wish to discharge herself for no apparent reason, might also have given a clue that something was wrong.

2 Heminevrin (Chlormethiazole) is a sedative drug which is itself addictive and therefore has to be given only over a short period of time and gradually reduced rather than suddenly stopped.

3 B and C.

4 Instead of total abstinence (never to take another drink) the patient may be a good candidate for controlled drinking under which he would be able to drink in definite moderation. This is achieved by helping him to learn to sip rather than to gulp, to have soft drinks in between spirits, to hold a conversation and be able to say 'no' when he wants no more, and to avoid the 'rounds' system, if necessary.

5 To answer this question, consider the gradual change in her behaviour, how she might get alcohol, diverting money from other purposes to pay for it, and the effect on her physical, psychological and social state.

Chapter 8   Self-evaluation

1 5%.

2 Overeating, secrecy, vomiting.

Chapter 9   Self-evaluation

1 Check the body of the text for your answers.

2 Instrumental.

3 Robbery with violence. The violence is in order to get money rather than just for the sake of violence.

4 Vicarious.

5 Prosocial aggression.

6 Competition or sport.

7 Behavioural contagion.
   Peer-group pressure.
   Overcrowding.
   Imitation.
   Subcultural expectation.
   To relieve frustration.

8 Assertive behaviour is that in which the individual asserts his own rights whilst respecting the rights of others. It is not designed to hurt in a physical or psychological way. The non-verbal communication accompanying the two behaviours is quite different.

Index

diazepam (Valium)   26, 48, 84
Diconal (dipipanone)   48
dieting   54–5
diet-related disorders   54–8
dipipanone (Diconal)   48
disulfiram (Antabuse)   53
dopamine   13
double-blind communications   14
drug dependence   9, 15, 46–7
   case history   50–2
drug induced abreaction   86
drug therapy   84–5
drug tolerance   47

electroconvulsive therapy (ECT; electroplexy)   85
environment, different, adaptation to   4
environmental factors   14–15
exhibitionism   72

fetishism   72
flupenthixol decanoate (Depixol)   84
flurazepam (Dalmane)   48
food   54
frigidity   71
frotteurism   72

glue abuse   49
groupwork/therapy   86

hallucination   44
haloperidol (Haldol; Serenace)   84
hashish (cannabis; marihuana)   46–7, 49
Heminevrin (chlormethiazole)   48, 84
heroin (diamorphine)   48
homosexuality   72
hospital addiction (Munchausen's syndrome)   25
Huntington's chorea   12–13, 39–40
hypnosedatives   48, 84
hypomania   29, 30–3
hypothalamus   61
hysterical neurosis   9, 24–5
      conversion reactions   24
      dissociative features   24–5

illness model   10
imipramine (Tofranil)   84
impotence   71
industrial therapy   88
infections   13
informal admission   20
insight   7, 15
institution, total   15–16

Jacob–Creutzfeld's disease   38–9

label   15
lanugo   56

Largactil (chlorpromazine)   84
learned helplessness theory   13
lesbianism   72
Librium (chlordiazepoxide)   48, 49
life events   14–15
lithium carbonate (Priadel; Camcolit)   85
lysergic acid diethylamide (LSD)   47, 49

mania   28
manic-depressive psychosis   9, 29–36
marihuana (cannabis; hashish)   46–7, 49
marriage   14
masochism   72
Mental Health Act 1983   19–22
   Commission   19
   compulsory detention   20–1
   informal admission   20
Mental Health Review Tribunal   21
mental illness   7–11
   causes   12–15
      biochemical   13
      cerebral   13
      genetic   12
   consequences   15–16
   definition   8
   World Health Organization classification   9
methadone (Physeptone)   48
methylphenidate (Ritalin)   49
milieu therapy   86
modified narcosis (sleep treatment)   26, 83
Mogadon (nitrazepam)   48, 84
mono amine oxidase inhibitors   84
mood-stabilizing drugs   85
morphine   48
motivation   5
multiple personality   25
Munchausen's syndrome (hospital addiction)   25
mushrooms, magic (hallucinogenic)   47, 49

Nardil (phenelzine)   84
necrophilia   72
neologism   44
neuroses   9
nitrazepam (Mogadon)   48, 84
noradrenaline   13
normality, definition of   8

obsessive–compulsive state (neurosis)   9, 25
occupational therapy   88
organizations   83

paedophilia   72
paranoid illness   9
parents   14
Parnate (tranylcypromine)   84
patients' different needs, adaptation to   4
personality   13–14